T0259382

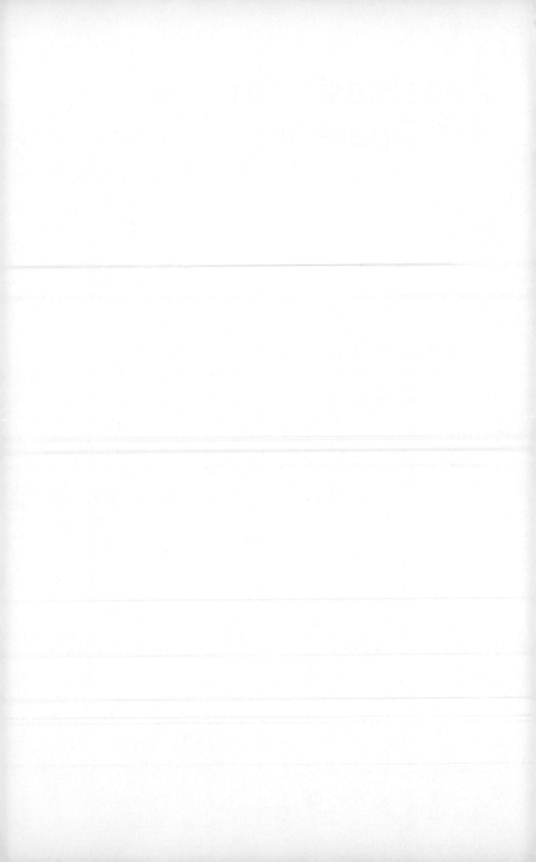

Anesthesia Outside the Operating Room

Guest Editors

WENDY L. GROSS, MD, MHCM
BARBARA GOLD, MD

ANESTHESIOLOGY CLINICS

www.anesthesiology.theclinics.com

Consulting Editor
LEE A. FLEISHER, MD, FACC

March 2009 • Volume 27 • Number 1

SAUNDERS an imprint of ELSEVIER, Inc.

W.B. SAUNDERS COMPANY
A Division of Elsevier Inc.

1600 John F. Kennedy Boulevard, Suite 1800 • Philadelphia, PA 19103-2899

http://www.theclinics.com

ANESTHESIOLOGY CLINICS Volume 27, Number 1
March 2009 ISSN 1932-2275, ISBN-13: 978-1-4377-0453-2, ISBN-10: 1-4377-0453-0

Editor: Rachel Glover
Developmental Editor: Donald Mumford

Anesthesiology Clinics (ISSN 1932-2275) is published quarterly by Elsevier Inc., 360 Park Avenue South, New York, NY 10010-1710. Months of issue are March, June, September, and December. Business and Editorial Offices: 1600 John F. Kennedy Blvd., Suite 1800, Philadelphia, PA 19103-2899. Customer Service Office: 6277 Sea Harbor Drive, Orlando, FL 32887-4800. Periodicals postage paid at New York, NY and additional mailing offices. Subscription prices are $122.00 per year (US student/resident), $244.00 per year (US individuals), $298.00 per year (Canadian individuals), $372.00 per year (US institutions), $461.00 per year (Canadian institutions), $172.00 per year (Canadian and foreign student/resident), $338.00 per year (foreign individuals), and $461.00 per year (foreign institutions). To receive student and resident rate, orders must be accompanied by name of affiliated institution, date of term, and the *signature* of program/residency coordinator on institutions letterhead. Orders will be billed at individual rate until proof of status is received. Foreign air speed delivery is included in all *Clinics'* subscription prices. All prices are subject to change without notice. POSTMASTER: Send address changes to *Anesthesiology Clinics,* Elsevier Periodicals Customer Service, 11830 Westline Industrial Drive, St. Louis, MO 63146. Customer Service (orders, claims, online, change of address): Elsevier Periodicals Customer Service, 11830 Westline Industrial Drive, St. Louis, MO 63146. Tel: 1-800-654-2452 (U.S. and Canada); 314-453-7041 (outside U.S. and Canada). Fax: 314-453-5170. E-mail: journalscustomerservice-usa@elsevier.com (for print support); journalsonlinesupport-usa@elsevier.com (for online support).

Reprints. For copies of 100 or more of articles in this publication, please contact the Commercial Reprints Department, Elsevier Inc., 360 Park Avenue South, New York, NY 10010-1710. Tel.: 212-633-3812; Fax: 212-462-1935; E-mail: reprints@elsevier.com.

Anesthesiology Clinics, is also published in Spanish by McGraw-Hill Inter-americana Editores S. A., P.O. Box 5-237, 06500 Mexico D. F., Mexico.

Anesthesiology *Clinics,* is covered in *MEDLINE/PubMed (Index Medicus), Current Contents/Clinical Medicine, Excerpta Medica, ISI/BIOMED,* and *Chemical Abstracts.*

Printed and bound in the United Kingdom
Transferred to Digital Print 2011

Contributors

CONSULTING EDITOR

LEE A. FLEISHER, MD, FACC
Robert D. Dripps Professor and Chair of Anesthesiology and Critical Care, University of Pennsylvania School of Medicine, Philadelphia, Pennsylvania

GUEST EDITORS

WENDY L. GROSS, MD, MHCM
Medical Director of Peri-Procedural Services; Cardiovascular Medicine Director of Non-OR Cardiac Anesthesia, Department of Anesthesia, Perioperative and Pain Medicine, Brigham and Women's Hospital, Boston, Massachusetts

BARBARA GOLD, MD
Associate Professor of Anesthesiology; Vice Chair, Education; Medical Director, University of Minnesota Medical Center, Minneapolis, Minnesota

AUTHORS

ANGELA M. BADER, MD, MPH
Associate Professor of Anaesthesia, Harvard Medical School; Director, Weiner Center for Preoperative Evaluation, Brigham and Women's Hospital, Boston, Massachusetts

RICHARD A. BAUM, MD
Division of Angiography and Interventional Radiology, Department of Radiology, Brigham and Women's Hospital, Harvard Medical School, Boston, Massachusetts

MAHESH BIKKINA, MD
Director of Cardiac Catheterization, Cardiac Intervention and Cardiac Research, St. Joseph's Regional Medical Center, Paterson, New Jersey

JASON P. CAPLAN, MD
Assistant Professor of Clinical Psychiatry, Vice Chair of Psychiatry, Creighton University School of Medicine, Omaha, Nebraska; Chief of Psychiatry, St. Joseph's Hospital and Medical Center, Phoenix, Arizona

PIERRE CASTHLEY, MD
St. Joseph's Regional Medical Center, Paterson, New Jersey

THOMAS W. CUTTER, MD, MAEd
Associate Professor and Associate Chairman, Department of Anesthesia and Critical Care, University of Chicago Medical Center, Chicago, Illinois

WILLEM J.S. de VILLIERS, MD, PhD, MHCM
Division of Digestive Diseases and Nutrition, Department of Internal Medicine, University of Kentucky Medical Center, University of Kentucky College of Medicine, Lexington, Kentucky

LUCY A. EPSTEIN, MD
Postdoctoral Clinical Fellow, Columbia University Medical Center, New York, New York

ROBERT T. FAILLACE, MD, ScM
Associate Professor of Medicine, Mt. Sinai School of Medicine; Chairman, Department of Cardiovascular Services, St. Joseph's Regional Medical Center, Paterson, New Jersey

REGINA Y. FRAGNETO, MD
Professor, Department of Anesthesiology, University of Kentucky College of Medicine, Lexington, Kentucky

ALLAN FRANKEL, MD
Principal Pascal Metrics Inc.; Faculty, Institute for Healthcare Improvement; Faculty, Brigham and Women's Hospital Division of General Medicine Patient Safety Group, Washington, DC

SAMUEL M. GALVAGNO, DO
Critical Care Fellow, Johns Hopkins University School of Medicine, Baltimore, Maryland

BARBARA GOLD, MD
Associate Professor of Anesthesiology; Vice Chair, Education; Medical Director, University of Minnesota Medical Center, Minneapolis, Minnesota

DANIEL T. GOULSON, MD
Professor; Director of Ambulatory Anesthesia, Department of Anesthesiology, University of Kentucky College of Medicine, Lexington, Kentucky

WENDY L. GROSS, MD, MHCM
Medical Director of Peri-Procedural Services; Cardiovascular Medicine Director of Non-OR Cardiac Anesthesia, Department of Anesthesia, Perioperative and Pain Medicine, Brigham and Women's Hospital, Boston, Massachusetts

ALEXANDER A. HANNENBERG, MD
Clinical Professor of Anesthesiology, Tufts University School of Medicine, Newton, Massachusetts

RAJA'A KADDAHA, MD
St. Joseph's Regional Medical Center, Paterson, New Jersey

NANCY M. KANE, DBA
Professor of Management, Harvard School of Public Health, Boston, Massachusetts

BHAVANI-SHANKAR KODALI, MD
Associate Professor, Harvard Medical School; Clinical Director, Department of Anesthesiology and Perioperative, and Pain Medicine, Brigham and Woman's Hospital, Boston, Massachusetts

RAMON MARTIN, MD
Department of Anesthesiology, Perioperative and Pain Medicine, Brigham and Women's Hospital, Harvard Medical School, Boston, Massachusetts

RUPEN PARIKH, MD
St. Joseph's Regional Medical Center, Paterson, New Jersey

MARGARET M. POTHIER, CRNA, BS
Department of Anesthesiology, Perioperative and Pain Medicine, Brigham and Women's Hospital, Boston, Massachusetts

JOHN QUERQUES, MD
Assistant Professor of Psychiatry, Harvard Medical School; Associate Director, Psychosomatic Medicine-Consultation Psychiatry Fellowship Program, Massachusetts General Hospital, Boston, Massachusetts

MYER ROSENTHAL, MD
Department of Anesthesiology, Stanford University, California

ROBERT M. SAVAGE, MD
Director, Perioperative Echocardiography, Departments of Cardiothoracic Anesthesia and Cardiovascular Medicine, The Cleveland Clinic Foundation, Cleveland, Ohio

MATTHEW P. SCHENKER, MD
Division of Angiography and Interventional Radiology, Department of Radiology, Brigham and Women's Hospital, Harvard Medical School, Boston, Massachusetts

DOUGLAS C. SHOOK, MD
Program Director, Cardiothoracic Anesthesia Fellowship, Department of Anesthesiology, Perioperative and Pain Medicine, Brigham and Women's Hospital, Harvard Medical School, Boston, Massachusetts

PAUL B. SHYN, MD
Division of Abdominal Imaging and Intervention, Department of Radiology, Brigham and Women's Hospital, Harvard Medical School, Boston, Massachusetts

RICHARD B. SIEGRIST, Jr., MBA, MA, BA, CPA
Adjunct Lecturer on Management, Harvard School of Public Health; President and CEO, PatientFlow Technology, Inc., Boston, Massachusetts

THEODORE A. STERN, MD
Professor of Psychiatry, Harvard Medical School; Chief, Psychiatric Consultation Service, Massachusetts General Hospital, Boston, Massachusetts

RICHARD TEPLICK, MD
Chief of Staff, University of South Alabama Hospitals; Associate Dean for Clinical Affairs, University of South Alabama College of Medicine, Mobile, Alabama

ANTHONY DUNSTER WHITTEMORE, MD
Chief Medical Officer; Professor, Department of Surgery, Brigham and Women's Hospital, Harvard Medical School, Boston, Massachusetts

THIL YOGANANTHAN, MD
Chief, Cardiac Anesthesia, St. Joseph's Regional Medical Center, Paterson, New Jersey

Contents

Achieving fundamental reform of the health care system to improve patient outcomes will take decades of effort and a major shift in financial, medical, and political behaviors that have built up since the beginning of health insurance in the United States. To the extent that the present payment systems contribute to the high cost, poor quality, and lack of accountability that characterizes today's health care delivery system, there is hope that reforms are within reach.

Most financial analysis regarding the cost of non–operating room anesthesia in hospitals is incorrect. This article indicates why this situation exists and suggests how to perform the cost analysis in the right way. It also reviews financial and operational strategies that can result in more efficient scheduling of anesthesia, thereby freeing up anesthesiologist time in the main operating room for non–operating room needs.

Modern invasive cardiovascular procedures require patients to be both comfortable and cooperative. In addition, these procedures demand the complete attention of the attending cardiovascular specialist, and, to a large degree, the outcomes of these procedures depend on the amount of focus and concentration the cardiovascular specialist can give to performing the procedure itself. A team approach using the specialized skills of a cardiologist and an anesthesiologist frequently is required to optimize results. This article clearly delineates the procedures cardiologists perform that might involve anesthesiologists. Mutual knowledge, understanding, and respect are fundamental requirements for integration of cardiology and anesthesia services to optimize patient outcomes.

Procedures and interventions in the cardiac catheterization laboratory (CCL) and electrophysiology laboratory (EPL) are more complex and involve acutely ill patients. Safely caring for this growing patient population in the CCL and EPL is now a concern for all anesthesiologists and cardiologists. Anesthesiologists are uniquely trained to care for this complex patient population, allowing the cardiologist to focus on completing the interventional procedure successfully.

A successful population-based colorectal cancer screening requires efficient colonoscopy practices that incorporate high throughput, safety, and patient satisfaction. There are several different modalities of nonanesthesiologist-administered sedation currently available and in development that may fulfill these requirements. Modern-day gastroenterology endoscopic procedures are complex and demand the full attention of the attending gastroenterologist and the complete cooperation of the patient. Many of these procedures will also require the anesthesiologist's knowledge, skills, abilities, and experience to ensure optimal procedure results and good patient outcomes. The goal of this review is (1) to provide a gastroenterology perspective on the use of propofol in gastroenterology endoscopic practice, and (2) to describe newer GI endoscopy procedures that gastroenterologists perform that might involve anesthesiologists.

Traditionally, sedation for gastrointestinal endoscopic procedures was provided by the gastroenterologist. Increasingly, however, complex procedures are being performed on seriously ill patients. As a result, anesthesiologists now are providing anesthesia and sedation in the gastrointestinal endoscopy suite for many of these patients. This article reviews the challenges encountered in this environment and anesthetic techniques that can be used successfully for these procedures.

Performing an anesthetic in a procedure suite instead of in the operating room can be extremely challenging for the anesthetist. Not only are the procedures performed outside of the operating room becoming increasingly more complex but also patient acuity is increasing. In some cases, the out-of–operating room procedure may be selected as a less risky alternative to an operating room procedure in an extremely high-risk patient. Effective preprocedure evaluation and preparation are critical to achieve optimal clinical outcomes and maximal operational efficiency in these areas.

The safety of anesthesia delivered in the operating room is enhanced by the standardization and reliability built into that environment, which has prescriptive and detailed protocols for almost every procedure performed. Experienced anesthesiologists come to rely on these operating room characteristics to support the delivery of safe care. Anesthesiologists giving anesthesia outside the operating room often find themselves in settings that lack this rigor and that therefore challenge safety. This article describes the basic concepts in safety, with an emphasis on teamwork and communication, and then discusses how their application ensures safe care in remote locations.

There is no need to reinvent the wheel to determine the need for vigilant monitoring in outside of the operating room (OOR) settings. Anesthesiologists have evolved a robust system of monitoring standards based on decades of experience in operating room environments. Every OOR location should be thoroughly evaluated and monitoring standards implemented. The standards should be periodically reviewed to avert morbidity.

Delivery of the spectrum of anesthesia from sedation to general anesthesia for patients undergoing procedures outside of the operating room (OR) poses several problems not encountered in the OR. These include limited time to assess the patient and often no time to obtain consultations for medical conditions that may be outside of the usual purview of an anesthesiologist, such as initial management of infections, diabetic ketoacidosis or hyperosmotic hyperglycemic state, inadequately managed cardiovascular disease, and toxic ingestions. Anesthesiologists trained in critical care usually have more experience with the initial assessment and management of patients with such conditions. It can be argued that because procedures performed outside of the OR are becoming more common, the curriculum for anesthesia residencies should be modified to provide more training in conditions typically assessed and managed by internists or medical subspecialists.

Whether we like it or not, medicine is big business. The argument is sometimes made that standard management strategies from the business world do not apply to medicine because the economics and practice of medicine are unique—driven by science and rapid rates of change. But an exploding knowledge base, light-speed technological development, and everchanging reimbursement schemes are *not* exclusive to medicine and health care. Some fundamental principles of finance, business management, and strategic development have evolved to deal with problems of rapid change. These principles do apply to modern medicine. The business side of anesthesia practice is off-putting to many clinicians. However, knowledge of the market forces at play can help enhance patient care, improve service, expand opportunities, and extend the perimeter of the discipline. The mission and current market position of anesthesiology practice are considered here.

THE CLINICS ARE NOW AVAILABLE ONLINE!

Access your subscription at:
www.theclinics.com

Foreword

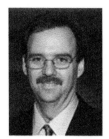

Lee A. Fleisher, MD, FACC
Consulting Editor

Increasingly, we are being asked to provide anesthesia or heavy sedation for patients undergoing procedures outside of the operating room. This represents a clinical, staffing, and financial challenge to most anesthesiology departments. While provision of anesthesia services within an operating room environment has been associated with increasing safety over the past several decades, settings outside of the operating room may present unique challenges. For these reasons, it is important the *Anesthesiology Clinics* address this important topic. In this issue, three major areas of care are addressed: financial implications, optimal care paradigms for specific patients, and locations and priorities with respect to all out-of-operating-room settings.

In choosing editors for this issue, it became important to identify forward thinkers from different locations to obtain a broad perspective of optimal care. Both Wendy Gross, MD, and Barbara Gold, MD, are such individuals. Dr. Gross is currently assistant professor of Anesthesia at Harvard Medical School and an attending anesthesiologist at the Brigham and Women's Hospital. She is currently the medical director of the Procedural Sedation Service and the Peri-Procedural Services in Cardiovascular Medicine and director of Non-OR Anesthesia Services at her hospital. Dr. Gold is currently associate professor of Anesthesiology and vice chair for Education at the University of Minnesota and medical director of anesthesia at Fairview Hospital. She has been a leader in the area of ambulatory anesthesia and a former president of the Society of Ambulatory Anesthesia. Together, they have produced an issue which will help us deal with new challenges in our practice.

Lee A. Fleisher, MD, FACC
Department of Anesthesiology and Critical Care
University of Pennsylvania School of Medicine
6 Dulles, 3400 Spruce Street
Philadelphia, PA 19104, USA

E-mail address:
fleishel@uphs.upenn.edu (L.A. Fleisher)

Anesthesiology Clin 27 (2009) xiii
doi:10.1016/j.anclin.2009.02.001   **anesthesiology.theclinics.com**
1932-2275/09/$ – see front matter © 2009 Elsevier Inc. All rights reserved.

Preface

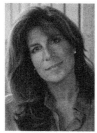 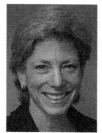

Wendy L. Gross, MD, MHCM   Barbara Gold, MD
Guest Editors

For the most part, anesthesiologists practice their specialty in the controlled setting of the operating room (OR). However, improved technology, escalating financial constraint, limited OR resources, and growing numbers of acutely ill patients create incentives for medical practitioners to perform procedures outside of the OR. Consequently, the need for deeper sedation, general anesthesia, and hemodynamic monitoring in non-OR venues has grown dramatically. In many hospitals, the non-OR caseload is equal to that of the OR. Many non-OR procedures are performed with minimal to moderate intravenous sedation administered by registered nurses, however, an increasing number require more extensive medications and regimens administered by anesthesiologists. Not only is the volume of non-OR cases increasing, but the scope of non-OR procedures requiring anesthesia care is increasing as well. This evolution generates new challenges for medical interventionalists, anesthesiologists, and patients alike.

As the practice of anesthesiology moves beyond the familiar domain of the OR, it enters the venue of medical specialists—such as invasive cardiologists, interventional radiologists, gastroenterologists, and oncologists. There are new obstacles to overcome as the landscape changes. The articles herein have been compiled to help the practitioner navigate the new landscape by examining the issues from multiple perspectives. This issue of *Anesthesiology Clinics* is divided into three sections, each of which scrutinizes the practice of anesthesiology in non-OR locations.

SECTION 1: FINANCIAL CONSIDERATIONS

This section discusses the context for major financial considerations that drive the practice of anesthesiology as it expands outward from the traditional perioperative area. These considerations include budget neutrality, new innovation, the cost of poorly integrated care, and financial implications of potential modifications to resource management in the OR. In the current reimbursement environment, anesthesia service

Anesthesiology Clin 27 (2009) xv–xvii
doi:10.1016/j.anclin.2009.01.002   **anesthesiology.theclinics.com**

provided outside of the OR is poorly reimbursed. Opportunity costs for anesthesia departments are enormous since coverage outside of the OR often requires a ratio of 1:1 staffing. The demand for comprehensive and reliable anesthesiology services outside of the OR is growing, but the benefits accrue to other departments and to hospitals as a whole. Just as surgical procedures in the OR often require an integrative and interdisciplinary approach to patient care and strategic management of reimbursements, so, too, do many of the emerging minimally invasive procedures performed outside of the OR. Creative financing and alternative staffing models may need to be considered.

SECTION 2: PRACTICE PARAMETERS

The authors review anesthesiology practice needs and methods as they evolve outside of the OR in three rapidly growing areas: cardiology, endoscopy, and radiology. Many non-OR procedures are new and innovative. Often, interventionalists perform novel procedures and employ new techniques that are unique or unfamiliar to them and to the anesthesiologists attending to their patients. Delivering anesthetic care to those who are acutely ill, elderly, and/or poorly prepared for the procedure is always challenging; performing this work during a procedure that is either ill-defined or poorly explained/communicated to the anesthesiologist adds another layer of complexity. A fundamental understanding of the types of cases performed and types of patients commonly treated in non-OR locations is critical.

Many non-OR areas have physical characteristics that are unwelcoming for anesthesiologists and their equipment. Often proceduralists are unfamiliar with the basic needs of anesthesiologists and the equipment needed to ensure patient safety. The necessary anesthesia equipment is usually expensive and may be incompatible with that of the interventional suite in terms of space or patient positioning. More importantly, sick patients require intense and complex anesthetic care even if the procedure itself is not complicated. Section 2 considers what medical specialists and anesthesiologists in cardiology, radiology, and endoscopy see as important practice guidelines and future goals for their respective practices.

SECTION 3: TRANSITIONAL PRIORITIES

Here, the authors discuss critical features of OR practice that must become standard in non-OR sites to insure consistency, patient safety, and best practice outside of the OR. The characteristics of consultative practice and the application of OR standards to non-OR locations are considered in this section. There is no question that anesthesiology stands at the forefront of promoting and developing increased patient safety. Perioperative morbidity and mortality have declined as anesthesia practice has evolved. In addition, surgical procedures have grown less invasive. Outside of the OR, however, the opposite is true. Whereas non-OR procedures were previously small and relatively simple, they are now as broad in scope as many surgeries, even though they may be less "invasive."

Percutaneous procedures often accomplish the same process and purpose as open surger. "Minimally invasive" percutaneous procedures introduce a different type of risk, however, because fixing a problem may be more difficult without exposure, necessitating urgent transfer of the patient to the OR. Nonsurgical practitioners may find it hard to understand why patients require invasive monitors or any monitors, or even the presence of an anesthesiologist until the unexpected happens in the middle of a procedure. In Section 3, the need for portability of standard OR practice parameters is discussed in terms of patient evaluation, monitoring, and safety.

In the final article, the future of anesthesiology as a medical specialty is discussed using the evolution of ICU practice as a template. In addition, strategies for the future are discussed in the context of emerging medical, political, and financial challenges. The future of the specialty now includes an array of practices in non-OR locations. We face the question of how to incorporate a new venue into the practice of anesthesiology and how to do so in a way that makes medical, political, and financial sense for the future of the specialty and medicine. The future of anesthesiology as a medical specialty is discussed. The financial and political challenges we face are summarized. An account of the new concerns we face, the changing practice parameters we encounter, and a review of what we know to be essential to the delivery of safe care concludes this issue. We discuss the need for our specialty to develop strategies that stimulate us to keep in step with the rhythm of modern medicine for the benefit of patients and practitioners.

Wendy L. Gross, MD, MHCM
Department of Anesthesia, Perioperative and Pain Medicine
Brigham and Women's Hospital
75 Francis St.
Boston, MA 02115

Barbara Gold, MD
Department of Anesthesiology
University of Minnesota Medical Center
Minneapolis, MN

E-mail addresses:
wgross@partners.org (W.L. Gross)
goldx002@umn.edu (B. Gold)

Introduction: The Challenge of Anesthesia Outside the Operating Room

Anthony Dunster Whittemore, MD

There is little doubt that the burgeoning array of minimally invasive procedures provides substantial advantages over traditional open surgical alternatives. Because significant complications have become low-frequency events, an aura of complacency is frequently notable in interventional suites. Yet such procedures, however minimally invasive they may be, are associated with potential hazard.

At the Brigham and Women's hospital in Boston, more than 30,000 operations are carried out annually in the setting of the conventional operating room, but an equal number of interventions are conducted in remote locations where the availability of anesthesia personnel is less predictable. This reflects a national trend with regard to the interventional endoscopy, radiology, and cardiology areas, most of which are associated with a low risk of anesthetic and procedural complications.

As the comorbidities of patients inevitably become more significant, however, the inherent risks of major cardiopulmonary complications, along with perforation and hemorrhage, remain real hazards. Patients are not always evaluated before non–operating room procedures with the standards or rigor insisted on for operating room cases. Anesthesia consults are often sought spontaneously at the last minute, or the need is not recognized at all. Practitioners administering sedation not infrequently provide inadequate analgesia and sedation for fear of inducing complications from overmedication; less frequently, respiratory distress or worse may occur. It is hoped that allocation of additional anesthesia resources results in a safer and more comfortable experience for patients and for all health care providers involved.

Department of Surgery, Brigham and Women's Hospital, Harvard Medical School, Boston, MA, USA
E-mail address: wgross@partners.org

Anesthesiology Clin 27 (2009) 1
doi:10.1016/j.anclin.2009.01.001
anesthesiology.theclinics.com

Introduction: The Challenge of Anesthesia Outside the Operating Room

SECTION 1:
FINANCIAL CONSIDERATIONS

Anesthesiology Clin 27 (2009) 3
doi:10.1016/S1932-2275(09)00026-3
1932-2275/09/$ – see front matter © 2009 Elsevier Inc. All rights reserved.

anesthesiology.theclinics.com

Introduction to Section 1: Financial Considerations

Alexander A. Hannenberg, MD

KEYWORD

- Procedural sedation

This section on financial considerations is intended to provide the tools and perspective needed to intelligently structure a service providing high-quality anesthetic care for patients undergoing procedures outside the traditional operating room environment. Dr. Siegrist's outline of analytic approaches to the cost of such services contains well-established principles and techniques that are essential to understanding and explaining the economic impact and requirements for this care. Dr. Kane's discussion of emerging payment issues should make the reader aware that "the times they are a'changing" and that models of payment for health care will evolve rapidly in an effort to cope with the affordability challenges.

It is fair to say that all the "W's" of traditional journalism (who, what, where, why, when, and how) are in flux with respect to procedural sedation and anesthesia. Anesthesia providers involved in gastrointestinal endoscopy procedures are living through the resulting turmoil. Last year's controversy surrounding Aetna's limitations on payment for anesthesia care during endoscopy[1] is an excellent example of the fundamental challenges faced by everyone involved in expanding the scope of anesthetic care outside the operating room. Left unsettled in this dispute are the key questions of who needs what kind of sedation administered by whom! When is anesthetic care medically necessary, and when is it a convenience for the patient or operator? The author estimates that if all endoscopy procedures in the United States were attended by an anesthesiologist, the total cost would exceed $5 billion annually at current rates. Such figures predictably will provoke a reaction like Aetna's, and providers must anticipate future demands from payers and purchasers.

There undoubtedly will continue to be a place for sedative administration by trained nurses. The range of settings and conditions in which these services are optimal will be debated. The role of anesthesiologists in setting standards and in training and clinically supporting these non-anesthesia providers will advance the quality, safety, and efficiency of the care provided. Who better to direct—at an institutional level and an individual patient level—the use of hypnotics, sedatives, and analgesics? The failure of the payment system to recognize this type of physician leadership creates an obstacle to building multidisciplinary teams to meet the growing needs in procedural sedation.

Newton-Wellesley Hospital, Newton, MA 02462, USA
E-mail address: ahannenberg@partners.org

Anesthesiology Clin 27 (2009) 5–6
doi:10.1016/j.anclin.2008.10.008
1932-2275/08/$ – see front matter © 2009 Elsevier Inc. All rights reserved.

anesthesiology.theclinics.com

These challenges are likely to provoke new models of payment, many of which are described in the article by Dr. Kane. In the Acute Care Episode[2] demonstration project, Medicare is revisiting bundled payments that lump together institutional and provider payments for certain orthopedic and cardiac procedures. In such models, the providers involved—rather than Medicare's fee schedules—make decisions about the value of each provider's contribution to the care of the patient. What judgments will they make, for example, about the anesthesiologist's service in the catheterization laboratory? These considerations clearly are uncharted territory but, just as clearly, will bring the physicians in touch with cost–benefit considerations from which existing payment systems substantially isolate them.

The emerging need to provide compelling evidence of the value of a professional service demands systematic aggregation of outcomes data and a steady stream of scholarly work to assess the justification, clinical benefit, and economic underpinnings of anesthesiologists' services, especially for those new to the clinical arena.

Boston, September 2008.

REFERENCES

1. Feder BJ. Aetna to end payment for a drug in colonoscopies. NY Times Dec 28, 2007. Available at: http://www.nytimes.com/2007/12/28/business/28.colon.html. Accessed December 11, 2008.
2. Centers for Medicare and Medicaid Services. Medicare Acute Care Episode Demonstration. Available at: http://www.cms.hhs.gov/demoprojectsevalrpts/md/itemdetail. asp?filterType=none&filterByDID=-99&sortByDID=3&sortOrder=descending& itemID=CMS1204388&intNumPerPage=10. Accessed November 10, 2008.

Traditional Fee-for-Service Medicare Payment Systems and Fragmented Patient Care: The Backdrop for Non–Operating Room Procedures and Anesthesia Services

Nancy M. Kane, DBA

KEYWORDS

- Medicare • Payment reform • Care fragmentation
- Bundling • Medical home

Medicare's traditional method of paying for units of service, be they hospital admissions, office visits, outpatient surgeries, or laboratory tests, evolved gradually from a payment system that originated in the 1930s, when private insurance for hospitalizations and physician services first emerged in this country. At that time, hospitals were just beginning to cure patients, emerging from their centuries-long primary function as almshouses that provided housing and minimal comforts to the sick poor. Desperate for capital resources, hospitals founded the first hospitalization insurance plans and designed their largely cost-based, open-ended payment systems to favor their own expansive growth. Physicians in the 1930s reluctantly joined private, largely physician-controlled insurance schemes to stave off compulsory public insurance. Fee-for-service was the payment system of choice for keeping insurers, with more restrictive or prescriptive forms of payment, out of the practice of medicine. Hospitalization and physician payment systems were designed to entice providers into accepting them, not to ensure that the right care was delivered at the right place and at the right time.

Harvard School of Public Health, 677 Huntington Avenue, Boston, MA 02115, USA
E-mail address: nkane@hsph.harvard.edu

Anesthesiology Clin 27 (2009) 7–15
doi:10.1016/j.anclin.2008.10.009   anesthesiology.theclinics.com
1932-2275/08/$ – see front matter © 2009 Elsevier Inc. All rights reserved.

TOO MANY PAYMENT SILOS

The delivery system has come a long way since the 1930s, when the hospital was the physician's private workplace. As capital costs and technological advances have accelerated, hospitals, physicians, and other health care providers, willingly or not, have become increasingly interdependent, but current payment systems and medical culture do not reflect these changed relationships. Medicare's 18 separate payment systems for 16 different provider/supplier types, plus two types of private insurance plan (medical and drug) represent an elaborate scheme of "silos" that frequently pits the interest of one set of providers (eg, physicians) against the interests of another (eg, hospitals), leaving the patient in a daze, looking for an ombudsman.

PROLIFERATION AND FRAGMENTATION IN THE SITES OF TREATMENT

Changes in the sites of treatment have exacerbated fragmentation. Medicare expenditures for inpatient care have fallen from 50% of total traditional (non–managed care) spending in 1996 to only 34.5% in 2006.[1] In the same decade, Medicare spending for outpatient care rose from 4.5% to 8.3% of total traditional spending, and spending for "other fee-for-service settings" including hospice, outpatient laboratory, ambulatory surgical centers, and health clinics, grew from 11.2% to 15.5% of total traditional spending. For surgical procedures, the shift from hospital-based to free-standing ambulatory surgical centers (ASCs) has been dramatic: Medicare payments to ASCs doubled between 2000 and 2006, and the number of ASCs increased by more than 50% to 4707. Surgical care runs the risk of increased fragmentation with the proliferation of hospitals specializing in cardiac, orthopedic, and general surgeries. The number of such specialty hospitals grew from 46 to 89 between 2002 and 2004 and reached 130 in 2006 after the 2004–2005 moratorium on new specialty hospitals expired.[2] Even within hospitals, new "noninvasive, nonsurgical" approaches to disease via radiology and medical specialty clinics increase the likelihood of fragmentation by adding a whole new cadre of providers with whom the patient and the primary care-giver must interact, often without an infrastructure for doing so.

INCREASE IN THE NUMBER AND TYPES OF PHYSICIANS INVOLVED IN PROVIDING SERVICES

Even within the same payment silo (eg, physician services), the scope and number of providers involved in specialty treatment has increased the need for better care coordination. Within imaging services, for example, where growth in units of service per beneficiary has exploded in the last decade, radiologists now receive 43% of Medicare payments; the rest go to cardiologists (25%), surgical specialties (9%), independent diagnostic testing facilities (8%), internal medicine (6%), and other specialists (10%).

The average Medicare beneficiary sees five physicians a year. Nearly two thirds of Medicare beneficiaries with three or more common chronic conditions (eg, coronary artery disease, congestive heart failure, and diabetes) see 10 or more physicians in a year.[3] Yet fewer providers than ever are willing to spend the time, much of it unreimbursed, to coordinate care or communicate with the patient or other providers regarding the implications of the various tests and procedures provided.

Because of fragmentation, lack of coordination, and the fee-for-service incentives of Medicare payment, there is enormous variation in resource use and adherence to recognized quality standards and outcomes within severity-adjusted episodes. For instance, for similar severity-adjusted hypertensive patients, a high-cost cardiologist in Boston spends 1.74 times more on evaluation and management, 1.56 times more on imaging, and 1.39 times more on tests than the average Boston cardiologist. Similar variation occurs across metropolitan areas: in 2002, physicians in Boston treating Medicare patients for hypertension used 96% of the national average resource use per episode, whereas physicians in Houston and Miami used 120%, and those in Minneapolis used only 87% of the national average. Clinical quality measures show similar variation within and across cities, and they are not correlated highly with relative resource use.

OVERPAYMENT OF HIGHER-TECHNOLOGY CARE AT THE EXPENSE OF LOW-TECHNOLOGY CARE

Besides paying in silos that fail to align incentives across provider types (eg, hospital and physician) or within provider types (eg, radiologist and cardiologist, or proceduralist and anesthesiologist), Medicare also has an imperfect process for recognizing the impact of new technology on treatment cost and outcome. This deficiency affects care delivery in at least two ways. First, payment recognition for new technology involving physician services lags behind the appearance of that technology by several years, thereby slowing its adaptation. Second, payment adjustments for new technology that has been disseminated fully into practice, with the associated improvements in technique and scale, also are slow in coming, leaving in place incentives to overprovide newer technologies at the expense of equally or even more effective alternative treatments. The rapid migration of technically intensive procedures from operating rooms to non–operating room areas under the auspices of competing nonsurgical medical practitioners has strained the capabilities of payment systems to keep up with the proliferation of new service sites and types of practitioners.

The Resource-Based Relative Value System (RBRVS) assigns weights to physician service units (eg, office visit, diagnostic test, surgical procedure) based on the relative costliness of the inputs used to provide services: physician work, practice expense, and professional liability expenses. The relative weights for roughly 6700 distinct services in the Health care Common Procedural Coding System, the coding system for outpatient care under Medicare, are supposed to be updated at least every 5 years to reflect changes in medical practice, coding changes, new data, and the addition of new services. The minimum lead time for a new code can be several years; for instance, it is 18 months for new laboratory tests, but the service must be already "widely used" before the American Medical Association's Current Procedural Terminology Committee that supervises the coding system for insurance billing will consider it. Thus a test may be in the market for up to 2 years before it even can be submitted.[4]

On the other hand, Medicare has been slow to adjust relative weights downward once a new technology is well integrated into practice. Thus input costs generally are higher in the early years (when physician work may be more intensive or longer per treatment, patients involved may be more severely ill, and/or equipment or supply expenses may be higher because of lower volumes) than in later years when the service is well established and is being applied in higher volumes to less severely ill patients. The relative weights, however, are not lowered automatically to reflect the reduced input costs. A sign that Medicare has not done a good job of adjusting for the "experience curve" and impact of volume on new technology is the number of codes whose relative weights are reduced in 5-year reviews, relative to those that are increased. In 1996, for the first 5-year review following the 1992 introduction of the RBRVS system, the Resource Use Committee (RUC) of the American Medical Association, responsible for recommending relative weight changes to the Centers for Medicare and Medicaid Services, recommended increased weights for 296 codes, no change for 650 codes, and decreased weights for only 107 codes. At the second 5-year review in 2001, the RUC recommended increased weights for 469 codes, no change for 311 codes, and decreases for only 27. The Centers for Medicare and Medicaid Services accepted more than 90% of the RUC's recommendations.[5]

Because adjustments to relative weights are budget-neutral within the physician payment silo, increases in payment weights distribute the "fixed" resources more into the higher-weighted services while reducing the share of the pie paid to lower-weighted services. This system creates very strong incentives (overpayments) for physicians to provide more services with higher relative weights (services with newer technologies) and to avoid providing services with lower relative weights (services that do not use new technologies, such as evaluation and management or care coordination).

This "fee-for-service-on-steroids" phenomenon is responsible, at least in part, for fueling the enormous growth in the volume of high-technology services provided to Medicare beneficiaries in recent years. Between 2000 and 2005, the cumulative volume of physician services per beneficiary increased 30%, with the greatest increases in imaging (61%) and tests (46%). These volume increases have fueled large, politically unpopular increases in Medicare Part B premiums and are largely responsible for the negative updates in the physician fee schedule that are required by current law. At the same time, evaluation and management services, which include vital but underprovided services such as care coordination and patient education, had the lowest per-beneficiary rate of increase over the 5-year period—less than 20%.

Relatively poor payment for coordination and other primary care services has contributed to a severe shortage of United States medical school graduates willing to enter primary care residencies.[6] Although foreign medical graduates have been willing to fill the gap in recent years, the difference in income between primary and specialty practice is growing, and this difference will aggravate a predicted shortage of primary care physicians just as the baby-boomers reach Medicare age with a host of chronic care needs.[7]

IMPROVING INTEGRATION OF CARE ACROSS AND WITHIN PAYMENT SYSTEMS: POTENTIAL REFORMS
The Problem of the Sustainable Growth Rate Formula Is Absorbing Policy Attention with no Remedy in Sight

Much of the recent policy debate about physician payment involves eliminating the Sustainable Growth Rate (SGR) constraint on physician fees. The SGR was imposed by Congress in the Balanced Budget Act of 1997, limiting growth in Medicare physician expenditures per beneficiary to inflation plus the per capita growth in gross domestic product using 1996 as the base year. Total physician expenditures have exceeded this limit since 2001, thereby mandating across-the-board cuts in physician fees since 2002. As of 2008, however, Congress has overridden its own mandate in all but one of the last 7 years; each delay in implementing the law creates an ever-deeper deficit to be recovered out of future years' physician expenditures. The cumulative SGR deficit has grown so large (more than $60 billlon as of 2007) that at least 9 years of 5% fee cuts each year would be needed to comply with the law. Trustees of the Medicare Trust Fund have called this projected series of negative updates "unrealistically low," but Congress has not yet come up with an alternative, budget-neutral way to address the problem. Meanwhile, the fees not cut do not keep up with inflation and encourage even greater volume growth, although the greater volume per beneficiary does not seem to be related to better outcomes or better patient satisfaction with care.[8] Finally, although the fee-for-service system strongly encourages more volume, which is not needed, it does not reward care coordination or high-quality care, which is urgently needed.

It is Time to Focus on Alternatives to Fee-for-Service in Provider Silos

Although there is some truth in the popular joke that the most expensive piece of technology in a hospital is the physician's pen, the reality is that other parties are encouraged by their payment systems to provide a greater volume of service without regard to quality of care, overall cost, or health care maintenance. Hospitals have strong incentives to admit patients and to increase the care they provide in the less constrained outpatient setting, as well as to discharge patients early. Postacute providers have strong incentives keep patients Medicare-eligible even if that means re-admitting them to acute hospitals for the requisite 3-day stay for conditions that otherwise might have been treated more effectively in a community-based or long-term care setting. Equipment and pharmaceutical suppliers are paid only if their products are used, so they engage in direct-to-consumer advertising and marketing campaigns directed at physicians. One of the biggest problems in traditional Medicare is that no one is held accountable for the quality or cost of the entire package of services delivered to a beneficiary during an episode of illness or a year of chronic disease. Worse still, no one is held responsible for keeping Medicare beneficiaries healthy.

The Medicare Payment Advisory Commission (MedPAC) has recommended to Congress a number of reforms that would begin to address provider accountability for services outside the provider's service and/or payment silo. Two of these reforms are described here, because they reflect the most recent discussions and recommendations to Congress in the spring of 2008. A third concept described here is not yet at the recommendation stage but is complementary to the other two. The three would represent significant change in the way delivery systems are structured and operated. Their potential impact, if enacted, could be much more far reaching than the 1983 payment reform that replaced retrospective cost-based reimbursement with prospective diagnosis-related group payments for inpatient care. That reform contributed to a 20-year decline in inpatient days (and related inpatient capacity), as well as to an explosion in the development and use of outpatient and postacute providers. Given the potential impact of these possible reforms, it is likely that their implementation, if passed, would take several years. Even with a phased-in implementation, however, it is likely that some institutions will adapt and thrive, and others will not.

Bundling Parts A and B for High-Cost, High-Volume Inpatient Admissions

MedPAC's April 2008 recommendation to Congress, unanimously adopted, reads as follows:[9]

> *To encourage providers to collaborate and better coordinate care, the Congress should direct the Secretary (of HHS) to reduce payments to hospitals with relatively high readmission rates for select conditions and also allow shared accountability between physicians and hospitals. The Congress should also direct the Secretary to report within two years on the feasibility of broader approaches such as virtual bundling for encouraging efficiency across hospitalization episodes. The Congress should require the Secretary to create a voluntary pilot program to test the feasibility of actual bundled payments for services around hospitalization episodes for select conditions. The pilot must have clear and explicit thresholds for determining if it can be expanded into the full Medicare program, or discontinued entirely.*

Under bundled payment, Medicare would pay a single entity (one in which all providers involved were represented) an amount that would cover the expected costs of providing all services for the hospitalization and related postacute period. This proposal could be implemented on a pilot/voluntary basis for organizations with an infrastructure already capable of receiving and allocating bundled payments. For those lacking such an infrastructure, a phased approach could include, first, a confidential information-only strategy and eventually incorporate mandatory bonuses and penalties within a fee-for-service withhold system ("virtual" bundling).

Bundled payment might begin by focusing primarily on holding hospitals, physicians, and postacute providers responsible for 30-day readmission rates, which vary from 13% to 24% depending on the state.[10] This plan would encourage hospitals to work with physicians and postacute providers to re-engineer the care process, addressing mortality, morbidity, readmission rates, and costs throughout the patient's hospitalization and recovery experience. A bundled payment system would encourage providers to do a better job of coordinating and communicating through hand-offs of patients through the process of care and across the traditional payment silos. Focusing on inpatient admissions as the trigger for bundling also targets the most costly Medicare beneficiaries; the most costly 20% of Medicare beneficiaries average 1.7 admissions per year.

Medical Homes

In the same April 2008 meeting, MedPAC Commissioners also unanimously supported the following recommendations to Congress:[10]

Congress should initiate a medical home pilot project in Medicare. Eligible medical homes must meet stringent criteria, including at least the following: Furnish primary care, including coordinating appropriate preventive, maintenance and acute health services; use health information technology for active clinical decision support; conduct care management; maintain 24-hour patient communication and rapid access; keep up to-date records of patient's advanced directives; have a formal quality improvement program; maintain a written understanding with beneficiary designating the provider as a medical home.

Medicare should provide medical homes with timely data on patient use. The pilot should require a physician pay-for-performance program. Finally, the pilot must have clear and explicit thresholds for determining if it can be expanded into the full Medicare program, or discontinued entirely.

Under a medical home arrangement, the designated provider would be paid a monthly capitation for providing comprehensive, continuous care and acting as a resource for helping patients and families navigate through the health system to select optimal treatments and providers. The provider would continue to be paid fee-for-service for providing Part B services, subject to a pay-for-performance component reflecting the provider's clinical quality and efficient use of resources. Specialists could qualify as a medical home when they sign up to manage specific chronic diseases of their patients, such as a cardiologist managing patients who have congestive heart failure, or endocrinologists managing the care of diabetics. The provider's efficient and effective use of resources ultimately would affect participation and payment levels in the medical home program.

Eligibility might be limited at first to beneficiaries who have at least two chronic conditions, and enrollment in a medical home would be voluntary. Beneficiaries still would be free to see specialists without a referral from the medical home, although they might have an obligation to inform the medical home of their use of a non–medical home provider. There would be no beneficiary cost sharing for medical home fees.

Medical homes would begin to address the fact that beneficiaries with chronic conditions do not receive recommended care and are sometimes hospitalized for events that could have been prevented with better primary care. Researchers have found that adult patients who have chronic conditions receive recommended care only 56% of the time.[11] Avoidable Medicare hospitalizations related to congestive heart failure, chronic obstructive pulmonary disease, hypertension, and three forms of complications for uncontrolled diabetes are among the top 12 reasons for Medicare hospitalizations.[12] One study found that 38% of patients without chronic disease experienced medical mistakes, that is, medication and laboratory errors caused by lack of coordination across care settings. Even more patients (48%) reported similar mistakes when four or more doctors were involved in their care.[13] Although medical homes will not solve all the problems caused by fragmentation, fee-for-service silos, and lack of incentives for physicians to work collaboratively to improve patient care, they at least are headed in the right direction.

Accountable Care Organizations

Although MedPAC made no recommendations to Congress regarding accountable care organizations (ACOs), the concept was discussed extensively as a means of controlling excessive volume growth and addressing the uneven quality of care provided to all Medicare beneficiaries, not just those who have chronic or acute conditions. An ACO would be a group of physicians, possibly including a hospital, that is responsible for quality and overall Medicare spending for their patients over the course of a year. It could involve fee-for-service payment with withholds, penalties, and bonuses, or could move into more bundled payment designs if an infrastructure is created to allocate payments across provider types. ACOs would be responsible for all patients within a geographic area who agree to participate, thus expanding the concept of bundling beyond medical homes and bundled hospitalization care to include well-care, prevention, and health maintenance. They could be voluntary groups of physicians who choose to work together or who are within the same hospital's primary service area, or they could be already established multispecialty group practices.

Many philosophical and practical issues regarding the implementation of ACOs remain to be worked out, ranging from whether they should be voluntary (in which case there could be selection bias) or mandatory (which would generate high resistance in many unstructured markets), whether they should include hospitals, and whether nonparticipating physicians would continue to have their fee updates subject to the SGR. The direction of the policy discussion clearly is to encourage broader provider accountability across the payment silos for patient cost, quality, and outcomes.

SUMMARY

The rising tide of uninsured and underinsured Americans is a sign that the health care financing system is broken. Many policymakers, providers, and beneficiaries, however, believe that the health care delivery system is broken, too. To the extent that the present payment systems contribute to the high cost, poor quality, and lack of accountability that characterizes today's health care delivery system, there is hope that reforms are within reach. Medicare, as the largest payer in the country, can lead the way, as it did with diagnosis-related groups and RBRVUs, to change fundamentally the dynamics of health delivery in the United States. Already private insurers are experimenting with care coordination, provider accountability, and pay-for-performance concepts on a smaller scale. Some are hampered in their efforts to distinguish high-cost and poor-quality providers effectively because of the relatively small numbers of patients per provider. Medicare could increase substantially the validity and credibility of the tools of provider accountability by combining its beneficiary population data and its technical expertise with those of private-sector insurers. The technical ability to identify episodes of acute and chronic illness and to link providers to clinical measures of care and outcomes is improving every day, making payment reforms linked to meaningful measures of performance increasingly possible.

The implications for providers are that payment incentives of the future are likely to favor care coordination; information systems; integration/collaboration across primary, inpatient, and postacute sectors; performance measurement; and re-engineered processes of care. Obviously a big challenge is timing; the old payment incentives to provide ever-higher volumes of care continue, and they continue to punish those who do "the right thing." Physicians seeking to maximize volume and intensity of services at the expense of appropriate, high-quality patient care will resist efforts to hold them accountable for outcomes such as readmissions and unexpected complications. Hospitals that fail to see the need to build a collaborative, interdisciplinary infrastructure that improves patient care across the silos will struggle along the same path that led to the demise of their predecessors who were unable to manage their lengths of stay in the 1980s. Forward-looking hospital systems already are experimenting with integrated physician–hospital care packages in the private sector (eg, Geisinger Health System's extended episode warranty on coronary bypass surgery)[14] and in Medicare Demonstration projects (eg, the Acute Care Episode demonstration project and the Hospital Gainsharing Project).[15] Achieving fundamental reform of the health care system to improve patient outcomes will take decades of effort and a major shift in financial, medical, and political behaviors that have built up since the beginning of health insurance in the United States. In retrospect, managing length of stay was a piece of cake!

REFERENCES

1. Medicare Payment Advisory Commission. Data Book. Washington, DC: Medicare Payment Advisory Commission; 2007. p. 9, 116, 118, 104. Available at: http://www.medpac.gov.
2. Medicare Payment Advisory Commission. Report to Congress specialty hospitals revisited. Washington, DC: Medicare Payment Advisory Commission; 2006. p. 4.
3. Medicare Payment Advisory Commission. Report to the Congress, increasing the value of medicare. Washington, DC: Medicare Payment Advisory Commission; 2006. p. 36, 107, 108.
4. Quinn B. Crossing the three chasms: complex molecular testing and Medicare regulations. Foley Hoag LLP, Boston.
5. Medicare Payment Advisory Commission. Report to the congress medicare payment policy. Washington, DC: Medicare Payment Advisory Commission; 2006, p. 142.
6. Bodenheimer. Primary care—will it survive? N Engl J Med 2006;355(9):861–4.
7. Tu HT, O'Malley AS. Exodus of male physicians from primary care drives shift to specialty practice: tracking report no. 17. Center for Studying Health System Change. Available at: http://www.hschange.org/CONTENT/934/. Accessed November 29, 2008.
8. Fisher E. The implications of regional variations in medicare spending. Part 2: health outcomes and satisfaction with care. Ann Intern Med 2003;138(4):273–87.
9. Meeting of the Medicare Payment Advisory Commission [transcript]. Washington, DC, April 9, 2008. p. 300–1.
10. Cantor JC, Belloff D, Schoen C, et al. "Aiming higher" results from a state scorecard on health system performance, commonwealth fund. Available at: http://www.commonwealthfund.org/publications/publications_show.htm?doc_id=494551; 2007; Accessed June 10, 2008.
11. McGlynn EA, Asch SM, Adams J, et al. The quality of health care delivered to adults in the United States. N Engl J Med 2003;348(26):2635–45.

12. Rich MW, Beckham V, Wittenberg C, et al. A multidisciplinary intervention to prevent the reasmission of elderly patients with congestive heart failure. N Engl J Med 1995;333(18):1190–5.

13. Schoen C, Osborn R, Huynh PT, et al. Taking the pulse of health care systems: experiences of patients with health problems in six countries. Health affairs web exclusive (not 3). Available at: http://www.healthaffairs.org. Accessed June 16, 2008.

14. Available at: http://www.nytimes.com/2007/05/17/business/17quality.html. Accessed August 12, 2008.

15. Available at: http://www.cms.hhs.gov/demoprojectsevalrpts/md/list.asp?listpage=2. Accessed August 12, 2008.

Financial and Operational Analysis of Non–Operating Room Anesthesia: the Wrong Way Versus the Right Way

Richard B. Siegrist, Jr., MBA, MA, BA, CPA

KEYWORDS

- Full costing • Differential costing • Non-OR anesthesia
- Management control • Operations management
- Queuing theory • Urgency classification • Scheduling

Most financial analysis regarding the cost of non–operating room (non-OR) anesthesia in hospitals is incorrect. This statement is strong, but this article indicates why this situation exists and suggests how to perform the cost analysis in the right way. It also reviews financial and operational strategies that can result in more efficient scheduling of anesthesia, thereby freeing up anesthesiologist time in the main OR for non-OR needs.

FULL COSTING—THE WRONG WAY FOR MOST DECISIONS

When performing cost analysis regarding non-OR anesthesia, most hospitals use a costing approach referred to as "full costing."[1] Full costing attempts to determine all the costs of a particular cost object, in this case anesthesia performed outside the OR, either in total (x dollars of anesthesia services provided to cardiac catherization) or per unit (anesthesia services provided to cardiac catherization at a cost of x dollars per catherization procedure). Full cost is measured as the combination of the direct costs for the cost object plus a "fair share" of the overhead of the institution.

Direct costs are directly traceable to or caused by the cost object, such as non-OR anesthesia services in the catherization laboratory, interventional radiology, ICU, or other unit. The direct costs of anesthesia services provided during cardiac catherization procedures typically would include the time of the anesthesia team, the supplies and drugs needed during the administration of anesthesia, and any specialized equipment devoted to cardiac catherization–based anesthesia.

Harvard School of Public Health, 677 Huntington Avenue, Boston, MA 02215, USA
E-mail address: rsiegrist@patientflowtech.com

Anesthesiology Clin 27 (2009) 17–23
doi:10.1016/j.anclin.2008.10.010

anesthesiology.theclinics.com

Indirect costs are not directly traceable to only one cost object and therefore must be allocated to multiple cost objects, using a reasonable allocation base such as salary dollars, square footage, or service hours. Typical indirect costs include the finance department, computer services, and administration. These indirect costs are allocated to other departments using the allocation basis and statistics for each department, employing either a step-down approach (in which a department can allocate costs only to those departments below it in hierarchical structure) or a reciprocal approach (departments can allocate cost to each other using simultaneous equations).[1]

Although full cost accounting is useful for indicating what non-OR anesthesia cost on a fully loaded basis and for external/regulatory reporting, it can be highly misleading for internal decision making involving non-OR anesthesia in matters such as expanding/contracting, adding/dropping, or making/buying. An example may help illustrate this analytical pitfall.

For example, assume that the cardiac catheterization laboratory requires 80% of an anesthesiologist's time and 80% of an anesthesia technician's time on an annual basis, and annually 1000 catheterization procedures require anesthesia. The full cost of a catheterization procedure with anesthesia is shown in **Table 1**.

This calculation is useful for establishing the cost for the anesthesia component of a catherization procedure, in this case $800 per procedure. This calculation, however, does not help show what the cost would be if the volume of catherization procedures requiring anesthesia increased by 10% (ie, 100 cases), whether money could be saved by hiring an outside anesthesia service to take over anesthesia support for the catherization laboratory, or if one catherization room should be closed if the volume of catheterizations dropped significantly. To answer these questions one needs to use the differential cost.

DIFFERENTIAL COSTING—THE RIGHT WAY FOR MOST DECISIONS

Differential costing compares how costs actually would change for the institution after implementation of a particular management decision.[1,2] In other words, differential costing shows how costs (and revenues) would change between situation A (often the status quo) and situation B (the proposed change). A 10% or 100-case increase in catherization volume requiring anesthesia support can serve as an example.

The full cost approach indicates that costs would increase by $800 per new procedure times 100 more procedures, or $80,000. In reality, the direct costs for anesthesia supplies and drugs would increase proportionately by 10% or $15,000 (10% of $50,000 + $100,000). Anesthesiologist and technician expenses would increase between

Table 1	
Analysis of the cost of anesthesia for a catheterization procedure	
Expense Item	**Cost in Dollars**
Anesthesiologist (80% of $300,000)	240,000
Anesthesia technician (80% of $100,000)	80,000
Anesthesia supplies	50,000
Anesthesia drugs	100,000
Total direct costs	470,000
Indirect allocations from step-down	330,000
Full cost in total	800,000
Full cost per unit ($800,000/1000 procedures)	800

0% and 10%, depending on whether they have available time, paid overtime would be incurred, or additional staff would be hired. Although more indirect costs may be allocated, a volume increase of 10% probably will not result in an increase in administration or information services. Accordingly, instead increasing by $80,000, the actual costs would increase by between $15,000 and $47,000 ($15,000 plus 10% of $240,000 + $80,000), depending on how costs actually change—a big difference that could lead to an incorrect decision if the full cost approach is used.

This example has illustrated how to use differential costing to evaluate alternative choices. More completely, the steps in alternative choice decision making are to

1. Define the problem
2. Identify the likely alternatives (usually including the status quo)
3. Evaluate the quantitative factors (how costs and/or revenues will change)
4. Evaluate the nonquantitative or qualitative factors
5. Make a decision[1]

For step #3, a common approach is to look at the specific differences between alternatives A and B in regards to revenue and costs, as follows:

Change in revenues (positive for increase, negative for decreases)
± Change in variable costs (positive for decreases, negative for increases)
± Change in fixed direct costs (positive for decreases, negative for increases)
± Change in indirect costs (positive for decreases, negative for increases)
= Net benefit/loss (positive for net benefit, negative for net loss)

This simple approach enables clinical and financial managers to analyze the impact on the organization of a variety of changes related to non-OR anesthesia.

This approach clearly involves a number of assumptions regarding how costs actually will behave if changes are made. These assumptions should be reasonable but do not have to be exact to make informed decisions. Each assumption can be tested using sensitivity analysis as follows:

- Would the decision change if the assumption changed by 10%? If so, that assumption should be investigated in more detail.
- Would the decision change if the assumption changed by 50%? If not, it is not necessary to spend any more time fine-tuning that assumption.

An alternative approach to sensitivity analysis is to determine how much an assumption could change before a decision would change; this determination indicates how comfortable the decision-maker is with that assumption.

POTENTIAL CONSEQUENCES OF INCORRECT DECISIONS

The beginning of this article indicated that most hospitals use the wrong information to make decisions regarding non-OR anesthesia. What are the potential implications of this oversight? First, the true incremental profitability of the expansion of services requiring anesthesia support usually is understated because under full costing the costs are overstated. This overstatement of costs may lead the institution to underinvest in new services or to limit the expansion of existing services that would make economic sense.

Second, the value of the anesthesia department to the institution may be understated because of the increased allocation of indirect costs to anesthesia as a result of increased volume when in fact those indirect costs will not increase because they are not differential. Third, negative incentives may be created for the anesthesia service because the department is held responsible for costs that it does not control, namely allocated indirect costs.

Finally, as demand for non-OR anesthesia continues to grow, administration may not recognize what additional personnel and non-personnel resources will be needed to meet that demand. In other words, the anesthesia department either will exceed budget and be criticized for justifiable increases or will be stretched thin with potential negative consequences for quality of care, staff satisfaction, and patient satisfaction.

ADDITIONAL QUESTIONS FOR DIFFERENTIAL ANALYSIS

Some of the additional pressing questions facing anesthesia could be addressed using differential cost analysis in conjunction with operations management:

- What would be the differential financial impact of devoting separate anesthesiologists or anesthesia technicians exclusively to non-OR anesthesia during certain times of the day or days of the weeks?
- What would be the differential financial impact of shifting certain services requiring anesthesia support from an inpatient setting to an outpatient setting?
- How can anesthesia scheduling be adjusted using queuing theory or simulation models to enhance productivity, staff satisfaction and profitability?

MANAGEMENT CONTROL IMPLICATIONS

Another important issue is the role anesthesiologists should play in this differential cost analysis and alternative choice decision making. Should the analysis be left to finance because of its expertise with numbers? The answer is a resounding no. Anesthesiologists usually are in a much better position to evaluate how things will change if a particular action is taken. Therefore, a joint effort or partnership between anesthesia and finance in performing the differential analysis will produce the most accurate results.

Once decisions are made, who should be accountable for the ultimate results? If anesthesia has been involved directly in the decisions and in formulating the assumptions and options regarding those decisions, anesthesia should be held accountable for the results. If, however, anesthesia is not involved to a significant extent, then anesthesia should not be held accountable for something not under its control. Holding someone accountable for something not under his or her control is a recipe for disillusionment at best and dysfunctional behavior at worst.[1]

MORE EFFICIENT USE OF ANESTHESIA RESOURCES THROUGH OPERATIONS MANAGEMENT

An important cost to any hospital is the inefficient use of expensive resources such as anesthesia. A common belief is that inevitably anesthesia resources will be underutilized frequently because of the complexity and unpredictability of the OR schedule, which dictates the use of anesthesia. This inefficient use of anesthesia resources can be reduced greatly through the application of operations management techniques, however.

In a normal OR situation, emergent/urgent cases wreak havoc on the productivity of the OR and anesthesia staff. Typically, emergent/urgent cases are handled in one of three different ways depending on the specific circumstances:

1. The OR schedule builds in holes during the day to accommodate emergent and urgent cases.

2. If a truly emergent case comes in and there is no hole to fit it in, an elective case is canceled or delayed to perform surgery on the emergent case.
3. Urgent but not emergent cases are delayed until the end of the day, after prime time.

These three ways of handling emergent/urgent cases builds in inefficiency from having holes in the schedule, creates physician/nurse/patient dissatisfaction and stress from bumping elective surgeries, and results in wait times (sometimes longer than clinical desirable) for urgent cases and boarding of these cases in the emergency department.

Anesthesiologists suffer from the unpredictability of the demand for their services (they may be called into an emergent case at any time), from the need to spend unplanned time after prime time to accommodate urgent cases at the end of the day, and from inefficient utilization resulting from the downtime created by holes in the elective surgery schedule. As a result, the operating room department (and accordingly anesthesia) typically operates at 70% to 75% utilization, but all the staff feel stressed because of the unpredictability.

The science of operations management offers a solution to this chaotic situation — the application of queuing theory to separate nonelective (emergent/urgent) from elective (scheduled) surgeries.[3] Nonelective cases, by their nature, are random in occurrence. One cannot schedule when the victim of an automobile accident will arrive for surgery or when a patient will present with a ruptured appendix. In contrast, elective surgeries are nonrandom and therefore are under the control of the hospital/surgery department through scheduling. When random and nonrandom patient flows compete for scarce resources (ORs, surgeons, anesthesiologists, nurses, and staff), unpredictability and inefficiency naturally result.

One solution that has been shown to be effective is to designate specific ORs on certain days of the week and certain times of the day for nonelective surgery only. Ideally, those ORs should be used only for nonelective cases, and all nonelective cases should be done in those ORs. Those ORs should be fully staffed and available when emergent/urgent cases arrive.

The number of ORs necessary for this purpose can be determined scientifically using priority-based queuing models and historical arrival patterns/case times of nonelective (emergent/urgent) cases. In this situation it is important to develop and apply rigorously a clinically based urgency classification system to determine case priority and maximum waiting times. For example, a truly emergent case that needs to be in the OR within 30 minutes of booking would be an "A" case, an urgent case that needs to be in the OR within 2 hours would be a "B" case, a case that clinically could wait 24 hours would be an "E" case, and so forth. These nonelective ORs should operate only at 40% to 60% utilization to accommodate the random arrival of emergent/urgent cases and the need to begin surgery within a clinically defined time period.

What are the benefits of having such nonelective ORs? First, waiting times for emergent/urgent cases typically decline by more than 20%, resulting in better patient care and a decrease in emergency room boarding. Second, OR time after prime time decreases significantly because urgent cases are done during the regular day, rather than after prime time. Third, elective cases rarely are delayed or canceled because of emergent/urgent cases, because those emergent/urgent cases are done in the nonelective rooms. Fourth, the elective OR rooms can be scheduled back-to-back with resulting utilization rates of 90% or greater. Even though the nonelective ORs operate at around 50% utilization, the overall OR utilization increases from 70% to 85% or more.

The ramifications of this separation of disparate patient flows potentially are enormous for anesthesia. First, the reduction in OR time after prime time means that the demand for after-hour anesthesia coverage is reduced substantially. Second, the increased prime time OR utilization means that anesthesia is used more effectively during the day, with lower downtime. Third, and most relevant for this article, anesthesia gains additional time to cover non-OR anesthesia needs with existing staff and existing resources.

The positive benefits described in this article can be illustrated best with a simplified example. This example assumes a hospital has 20 ORs and currently is operating at a 70% utilization rate during prime time. Looking at emergent/urgent arrival rates and case times and applying queuing theory, the hospital determines that two ORs should be designated as nonelective ORs, and the remaining 18 ORs should be used only for elective cases.

Table 2 shows the freed-up capacity that is available for (1) moving cases done past prime time into prime time, (2) accommodating new surgical cases if demand exists, or (3) reducing OR staffing needs while handling the same number of cases.

In effect, such a change would enable the hospital to increase its surgical volume by 23% without adding any additional OR or anesthesia staff or any expenditure for new capital expenses. This increase in capacity results from improving the utilization rate from 70% to 86% (18 elective rooms at 90% utilization because of back-to-back scheduling of elective cases plus two nonelective rooms at 50% utilization to reduce wait times for emergent/urgent cases equals 86% overall utilization).

More relevantly to non-OR anesthesia, this change could free up 19% of anesthesia time normally spent in the OR for performing anesthesia in other settings. This reduction in staffed rooms for anesthesia results from needing to staff only 16.3 rooms to accommodate the existing volume of surgery (20 rooms at 70% utilization is mathematically equivalent to 16.3 rooms at 86% utilization in terms of surgical capacity). In most institutions this extra capacity probably would go a long way in addressing the chronic shortage of anesthesia resources for demands outside the OR.

This analysis makes the implicit assumption that the demand for elective surgery is relatively stable across the days of the week and that none of the low utilization can be attributed to variations in utilization across the days of the week. Accordingly, to achieve fully the benefits described in this example, an institution also would need

Table 2
Management of cases before and after dedicating two operating rooms for emergent cases

Metric	Comparison	Elective Rooms	Non-Elective Rooms	Total
Number of staffed rooms	Before	20	0	
	After	18	2	
Operating room utilization (prime time 7:30–3:30)	Before	70%	0%	70%
	After	90%	50%	86%
Occupied rooms	Before	14.0	0.0	14.0
	After	16.2	1.0	17.2
Difference		2.2	1.0	17.2
Increase in capacity				23%
Number of staffed rooms needed if assume no increase in prime-time surgeries	Before	20	0	20
	After	14.3	2	16.3
Reduction in staffed rooms				19%

to work on smoothing surgical demand across the days of the week by adjusting block schedules and taking into account destination unit capacity for inpatient surgeries.

Because the elective schedule is under the control of the hospital/surgery department, it should be possible to accomplish this smoothing of surgical demand with the cooperation of the surgeons. The benefits to the hospital, the nurses, the anesthesiologists, the surgeons, and the patients should be compelling enough to bring about these operational changes.

These improvements in utilization can translate into a significant opportunity for increased revenue and profitability. A 23% growth in surgical volume with no incremental staffing or capital costs related to OR or anesthesia equates to millions of dollars of additional profitability for the hospital, the surgeons, and the anesthesiologists. Applying the differential costing techniques described earlier makes quantifying these benefits feasible.

In summary, the marriage of cost accounting and operations management can help the anesthesia department (1) understand the true differential cost and benefits of non-OR anesthesia and (2) free up anesthesia resources for use in non-OR settings. The arguments for proper cost accounting, operations management, and optimized utilization in the OR apply with equal validity to the non-OR setting. Elective and emergent scheduling should be handled in the non-OR environment the same way that it is handled in the OR. Understanding how to apply differential cost analysis and queuing theory are the keys to making the right management decisions for the ORs, for procedure areas, and for the organization.

REFERENCES

1. Anthony RN, Young DW. Management control in nonprofit organizations. 7th edition. New York: McGraw Hill Irwin; 2003. p. 221–43, 272–95, 372–96.
2. Anthony RN, Welsch GA. Fundamentals of management accounting. 3rd edition. Homewood (IL): Richard D. Irwin; 1981. p. 246–62.
3. Litvak E, Long MC, Prenney B, et al. Improving patient flow and throughput in California hospitals operating room services. Boston university program for management of variability in health care delivery. California Healthcare Foundation 2007. Available at: http://www.bu.edu/mvp/Library/CHCF%20Guidance%20document.pdf.

SECTION 2:
PRACTICE PARAMETERS

Anesthesiology Clin 27 (2009) 25
doi:10.1016/S1932-2275(09)00025-1
1932-2275/09/$ – see front matter © 2009 Elsevier Inc. All rights reserved.

anesthesiology.theclinics.com

Introduction to Section 2: Practice Parameters

Barbara Gold, MD

The need for non-operating room (OR) anesthesia services continues to expand as technology improves and the scope of procedures performed by cardiologists, radiologists, gastroenterologists, and other physicians grows. Indeed, the range of procedures that can now be performed safely and comfortably outside the OR is facilitated by many factors, not the least of which are improvements in sedation and anesthesia care. However, each of these non-OR settings has different needs and limitations.

Delivering anesthesia in an operating room is a consistently structured endeavor irrespective of the specialty; a given OR can accommodate a wide variety of cases ranging from urologic surgery to neurosurgery. This is not the case in the non-OR setting; delivering anesthesia in a GI suite is qualitatively different than doing so in a cardiac catheterization lab—equipment is highly specialized, patient comorbidities are often unique to the particular specialty, physical access to the patient may vary, and the "culture" of the venue may make integration and communication difficult. For example, in the cardiac catheterization or EP lab, imaging equipment is often permanently affixed at the head of the bed, precluding easy access to the patient's airway. Given the myriad screens and equipment around patients, there may be inadequate space for anesthesia equipment, especially when tables move to permit fluoroscopy. There may also be confusion as to the handling of lab specimens as well as communication of lab results to anesthesiologists if there is no standard protocol. Again, coping with these situations may be straightforward in an OR setting; outside the OR, however, basic work processes cannot be assumed.

Work spaces are frequently retrofitted to accommodate anesthesia providers (and associated equipment) because procedural areas were not constructed with anesthesia delivery in mind. This often produces less-than-ideal working conditions for the anesthesia team. For example, medical specialists often dim ambient lights to accommodate digital images, making it difficult for the anesthesiologist to see equipment or observe patients. In addition, moribund patients deemed too sick to undergo an operation are often scheduled for a more limited procedure that nevertheless requires an anesthetic. The mix of unfamiliar work environment and processes along with a moribund patient can be especially problematic. However, anesthesia providers can help improve their work environment by becoming involved in the design phase of procedural facilities and also establishing working relationships with the subspecialty physicians. Indeed, as facilities are remodeled to accommodate the growing number of complex procedures performed outside the traditional confines of the OR, subspecialists increasingly are seeking the input of anesthesia care providers.

Department of Anesthesiology, University of Minnesota Medical Center, Minneapolis, MN, USA

Anesthesiology Clin 27 (2009) 27–28
doi:10.1016/j.anclin.2008.12.001   anesthesiology.theclinics.com
1932-2275/08/$ – see front matter

Due to the complex nature of the procedures and the fragile state of many patients, it is incumbent upon anesthesia providers to agree upon the "terms of engagement" in non-OR settings before providing actual patient care. That is, the provision of equipment, space, support services, and patient access needs to be addressed in detail and as far in advance as possible. Those working with fragile patients will further appreciate the need to address these issues as they learn about highly complex procedures that are just on the horizon, such as those described by DeVilliers (ie, natural orifice transluminal endoscopic surgery) or Faillace (ie, percutaneous ventricular assist devices).

This section explores major non-OR procedures that require anesthesia services from the vantage points of *both* the subspecialist performing the procedure and the anesthesiologist. Areas of convergent and divergent opinion are quite clear, and it is obvious that although the goals of both teams are similar, the focus of attention is not. The potential for expanding procedures outside the OR appears exciting and limitless, but the path to success requires both medical and diplomatic flexibility. The nature of these procedures and their associated patient populations (ie, older, medically compromised) could broaden the practice of anesthesiology and take our specialty in another exciting, challenging, and rewarding direction.

The Role of the Out-of-Operating Room Anesthesiologist in the Care of the Cardiac Patient

Robert T. Faillace, MD, ScM*, Raja'a Kaddaha, MD, Mahesh Bikkina, MD, Thil Yogananthan, MD, Rupen Parikh, MD, Pierre Casthley, MD

KEYWORDS

- Anesthesia • Invasive cardiology • Conscious sedation
- State-of-the-art cardiac interventions

Modern invasive cardiovascular procedures require patients to be both comfortable and cooperative. In addition, these procedures demand the complete attention of the attending cardiovascular specialist. To a large degree, outcomes of procedures depend on the amount of focus and concentration the cardiovascular specialist can give to performing the procedure itself. A team approach using the specialized skills of a cardiologist and an anesthesiologist frequently is required to optimize results.

At present there are no established, discipline-directed guidelines for anesthesia consultation or conscious sedation during cardiovascular procedures. The goals of the cardiologist in involving an anesthesiologist during the performance of cardiovascular procedures are to minimize physical discomfort, pain, and negative psychologic response to treatment; to ensure some degree of amnesia; to gain the patient's cooperation; to have minimal variation in the hemodynamic state; and to return the patient to a state in which safe discharge is possible.[1]

It is important that patients who have comorbidities that increase the risk associated with conscious sedation be recognized and assessed properly before initiating the procedure. The goal is to avoid complications during the procedure, especially complications related to maintenance of the patient's airway and hemodynamic stability. Patients at high risk include those who have morbid obesity, obstructive sleep apnea, chronic obstructive lung disease, congestive heart failure, hemodynamic compromise, an American Society of Anesthesia type III airway, and those taking medications that complicate their sedation/anesthesia requirements. The selection of medications used for conscious sedation/general anesthesia depends on the specific needs of the patient

St. Joseph's Regional Medical Center, 703 Main Street, Paterson, NJ 07503, USA
* Corresponding author.
E-mail address: faillacert@hotmail.com (R.T. Faillace).

Anesthesiology Clin 27 (2009) 29–46
doi:10.1016/j.anclin.2008.10.006   anesthesiology.theclinics.com

and on the complexity and duration of the procedure. Therefore, cardiologists and anesthesiologists need to have mutual understanding, common knowledge, and non-negotiable mutual respect to work together as a team to provide optimal care to the patient.

Common diagnostic and therapeutic invasive procedures performed by cardiologists fall under the domain of the cardiac catheterization laboratory, the electrophysiology laboratory, and the transesophageal echocardiography (TEE) laboratory. Specific procedures performed in the cardiac catheterization laboratory or electrophysiology laboratory that may benefit from the presence of an anesthesiologist include

Diagnostic cardiac catheterization
Percutaneous coronary interventions (PCIs)
Peripheral vascular diagnostic and therapeutic procedures
Use of percutaneous left ventricular assist devices for hemodynamic support in the setting of cardiogenic shock and/or high-risk coronary interventions
Placement of septal device occluders
Radiofrequency ablation procedures
Implantation of biventricular pacing systems and cardioverter defibrillators; and electrical cardioversion; percutaneous cardiac valve-related procedures

In addition, the performance of TEE may benefit from the input of an anesthesiologist, because it involves airway manipulation.

This article clearly delineates the procedures cardiologists perform that might involve anesthesiologists. Close collaboration between the cardiovascular specialist and the anesthesiologist is a fundamental requirement to optimize patient outcomes.

PROCEDURES PERFORMED IN THE CARDIAC CATHETERIZATION LABORATORY

It is estimated that more than 2 million Americans will undergo coronary arteriography with left ventriculography in the United States this year alone.[2] Diagnostic cardiac catheterization is performed to assess the presence and severity of suspected underlying cardiac disease that cannot be evaluated sufficiently by noninvasive techniques.[3] These conditions include coronary artery disease, valvular heart disease, congenital heart disease, and cardiomyopathic disease.[4] Cardiac catheterization laboratory–based procedures most commonly include left and right heart catheterization with hemodynamic measurements, left ventriculography with use of radio-iodinated contrast medium, diagnostic coronary arteriography, and PCIs. Diagnostic cardiac catheterization also may include the use of intracoronary ultrasound to assess the severity of luminal narrowing caused by an atherosclerotic plaque.[5] Patients who undergo cardiac catheterization range from hemodynamically stable outpatients to critically ill and hemodynamically unstable patients who have acute myocardial ischemia, severe heart failure, or cardiogenic shock.[3,6] The invasive cardiologist most commonly administers conscious sedation for hemodynamically stable patients. However, patients who are either critically ill, high risk, morbidly obese or patients who have severe obstructive sleep apnea, advanced underlying pulmonary disease are in need of complex prolonged interventions benefit from the presence of an anesthesiologist.

Percutaneous Coronary Interventions

PCIs include coronary angioplasty, coronary stenting with use of either bare-metal stents or drug-eluting stents, and atherectomy procedures. Percutaneous interventional procedures commonly are performed on patients who have demonstrated myocardial ischemia and 70% or greater intracoronary luminal obstruction from coronary atherosclerosis. The major benefit of PCI is to reduce or relieve symptoms and signs of ischemic heart disease.[7] In unstable patients or in patients who have ST elevation myocardial infarction, PCI may decrease mortality and subsequent myocardial infarction more effectively than medical treatment.[8–10] In patients who have stable coronary artery disease, however, a recent large, multicentered study has suggested there are no significant differences in total mortality, nonfatal myocardial infarction, and rate of hospitalization for acute coronary syndrome between patients randomly assigned to aggressive medical therapy or to aggressive medical therapy or bare-metal stenting.[11] To the authors' knowledge, no randomized trials have compared aggressive medical therapy alone versus aggressive medical therapy plus drug-eluting stents.

More recently, there has been an increase in PCIs and a concomitant decrease in coronary artery bypass graft surgery for unprotected (in the absence of coronary artery bypass grafts to the left anterior descending and left circumflex-marginal system) left main coronary artery disease.[12] Although at present at least five ongoing randomized, controlled trials with an anticipated enrollment of more than 2400 patients are comparing PCI and coronary artery bypass graft surgery for the treatment of unprotected left main coronary artery disease, no randomized study data have been reported as yet.[13] A recent meta-analysis of 16 observational studies involving 1278 patients undergoing PCI with drug-eluting stents for unprotected left main coronary artery disease demonstrated mortality of 2.3% during hospitalization and 5.5% at a median of 10 months' follow-up.[14] A recent registry study conducted in Korea in matched cohorts of patients who had unprotected left main coronary artery disease followed on average for 3 years demonstrated no difference in either death or a composite outcome of death, Q-wave myocardial infarction, and/or stroke for patients who underwent either PCI (with bare metal or drug-eluting stents) or coronary artery bypass graft surgery.[15] Target-vessel revascularization was significantly higher in patients who received stents (hazard ratio, 4.76; 95% confidence interval, 0.75–1.62), however.[15] This study also demonstrated a trend toward higher rates of death and the composite end point of death, Q-wave myocardial infarction, and/or stroke in patients who received a drug-eluting stent than in patients who received a bare-metal stent.[15] This study further shows the need for a adequately powered prospective, randomized trial of the two revascularization strategies in this population of patients.[13]

Cardiac catheterization and PCI procedures are performed most commonly with conscious sedation. In these patients the goal is to achieve a state of relaxation, analgesia, and amnesia that allows a patient to respond appropriately to verbal commands and maintain a patent airway. It is imperative that patients be able to cough immediately after the injection of radio-iodinated contrast medium into the coronary arteries to increase intrathoracic pressure and clear the dye from the arteries and prevent complications of myocardial ischemia and bradycardia.

Although in the authors' experience the invasive/interventional cardiologist administers conscious sedation for most diagnostic cardiac catheterization and PCI procedures, the need for an anesthesiologist becomes greater as the patient complexity, comorbidities and the procedural difficulty increase. These procedures may involve patients who have chronic total coronary artery occlusions, saphenous vein PCI interventions, or in-stent restenosis or patients who have complex coronary anatomy, are hemodynamically compromised, or who are in cardiogenic shock. In addition, patients who undergo PCI atherectomy procedures typically have more complex anatomy that requires the full attention of the interventional cardiologist. Atherectomy procedures also are time consuming. Rotational atherectomy uses a rapidly rotating, diamond-coated, olive-shaped burr and has been found to be useful for heavily calcified complex lesions. The burr pulverizes the atherosclerotic plaque into pieces small enough to pass through the distal myocardial capillary bed.[16] One uncontrolled, multicenter registry study demonstrated that this technique successfully relieved the luminal coronary artery obstruction in 94% of calcific lesions.[17]

Percutaneous Ventricular Assist Devices

Although intravenously administered positive inotropic medications and an intra-aortic counterpulsation balloon are used routinely to support a failing heart, more recent procedures performed in the cardiac catheterization laboratory include use of percutaneously placed left ventricular support devices. These devices support patients who are at high risk for a PCI procedure (eg, a patient with an unprotected left main lesion), patients who are hemodynamically compromised, and patients in cardiogenic shock. Two percutaneous ventricular assist devices currently are available clinically, the TandemHeart (Cardiac Assist, Inc., Pittsburg, Pennsylvania) and the Impella Recover LP 2.5 and 5.0 (Abiomed Inc., Danvers, Massachusetts).[18–20] The TandemHeart is used more frequently to support patients in cardiogenic shock (until a recovery occurs or as a bridge to definitive therapy) or as a temporary hemodynamic support during high-risk angioplasties.[19] The TandemHeart is a percutaneously placed left atrial-to-femoral bypass system. It comprises a transseptal cannula, arterial cannulae, and an externally located centrifugal blood pump. At a maximum speed of 7500 rpm, the pump can deliver flow rates up to 4.0 L/min.[19] One center reported a 30-day survival rate of 61% in 18 patients (11 in cardiogenic shock and 7 undergoing high-risk PCI) with use of the TandemHeart device. The cardiac index of patients in cardiogenic shock improved from 1.57 L/min/m2 before support to 2.60 L/min/m^2 with use of the device.[19] The mean duration of support was 88 ± 74.3 hours (range, 4–264 hours). High-risk patients undergoing PCI were supported by the device from 1 to 24 hours (mean 5.5 ± 8.3 hours).[19]

The Impella Recover LP 2.5 and 5.0 pump devices are similar percutaneous-based left ventricular assist devices.[21] One main difference between the Impella systems and the TandemHeart is that the Impella Recover LP 2.5 and 5.0 pump systems use cannulae retrogradely inserted via the femoral artery into the left ventricle across the aortic valve.[22] The main advantages of the Impella Recover LP 2.5 and 5.0 devices, as compared with the TandemHeart, are their ease of implantation, avoidance of the need for a transseptal puncture, and smaller catheter size (13 F versus 17 F). In addition, the microaxial pump is integrated directly into the catheter system, and there is no extracorporeal blood. The circulatory support of the Impella is either 2.5 L/min or 5.0 L/min. Patients must be selected carefully, because the Impella Recover LP 2.5 device requires the presence of at least some left ventricular function, whereas the TandemHeart device may replace left ventricular function completely.[22]

Patients who require use of either the TandemHeart or the Impella LP 2.5 devices definitely benefit from the services of a cardiac anesthesiologist. These patients are at high risk for either a morbid or life-threatening event during the procedure. The anesthesiologist and the cardiovascular specialist need to maintain adequate conscious sedation or general anesthesia and an adequate hemodynamic state. In addition, although preliminary reports have not cited any major adverse effects from the use of either device, cardiac surgical backup should be available during the performance of these procedures, because significant blood loss may occur.[23]

Percutaneous Closure of Septal Defects

Another procedure that would benefit from the presence of a cardiac anesthesiologist is placement of an intra-atrial septal occluder device for the treatment of either a patent foramen ovale (PFO) or an atrial septal defect. In 2001 the Food and Drug Administration (FDA) approved two occluder devices, the CardioSEAL Septal Occlusion system

(NMT Medical, Inc., Boston, Massachusetts) and the AMPLATZER Septal Occluder (AGA Medical Corporation, Golden Valley, Minnesota).[24] Other devices that currently are available include the Helex implant (W.L. Gore & Associates, Flagstaff, Arizona); the Premere PFO Closure System (St. Jude Medical, Inc., Maple Grove, Minnesota); the Solysafe Septal Occluder (Swiss Implant AG, Solothurn, Switzerland); the Intrasept occluder (Cardia, Inc., Burnsville, Minnesota); the Occlutech device (Occlutech, Jena, Germany), the SeptRx Occlude (Secant Medical, Perkasie, Pennsylvania); the BioSTAR septal occluder (NMT Medical), the first partially bioabsorbable septal repair implant; the SuperStitch device (Sutura(R) Inc., Fountain Valley, California); and the PFx Closure System (Cierra, Inc., Redwood City, California). The PFx Closure System uses vacuum suction to hold the septum primum and secundum in place and radio-frequency energy to close the PFO.[25] Despite this plethora of available devices, there has not been a prospective, randomized, controlled trial of percutaneous closure of PFOs in patients who have suffered from a cryptogenic stroke. In addition, no device has been approved by the FDA for the prevention of recurrent cryptogenic stroke.[26] Here the authors describe the AMPLATZER and the CardioSEAL devices because they are used commonly to close PFOs and atrial septal defects.

The AMPLATZER Septal Occluder consists of a percutaneous-based delivery system and a two-sided permanent occluder implant that resembles a clamshell.[26] The AMPLATZER Septal Occluder clamshell consists of two flat discs with a middle or "waist." The discs are made of nitinol (an alloy of nickel and titanium) wire mesh with polyester fabric inserts. These fabric inserts help close a patent foramen ovale or an atrial septal defect while providing a foundation for the growth of tissue over the occluder after placement.[27] It is claimed that the AMPLATZER Septal Occluder has several advantages over other devices, including delivery through smaller catheters; easy repositioning with a self-centering mechanism; a smaller overall size; and round retention discs extending radially beyond the defect that allow firmer contact and thereby enhance endotheliazation that, in turn, reduces the risk of residual shunting.[28]

The CardioSEAL device consists of two self-expanding Dacron-covered umbrellas that attach to either side of the intra-atrial septum. The umbrellas are formed by four radiating metal arms attached in the center. Because of arm fractures and protrusion of the arm through the atrial septal defect, the device was re-engineered by adding a self-centering mechanism made of nitinol springs. These springs connect the two umbrellas and a flexible core wire with a pin-pivoting connection. This device, named the "STARFlex," has reduced the rate of arm fractures significantly.[29,30]

Although the FDA initially approved these devices for percutaneous closure of secundum atrial septal defect in 2001, this approval was under the auspices of a humanitarian device exemption (HDE). This HDE was withdrawn in October 2006 because the devices were placed in more than 4000 patients, the limit set by the FDA.[31] Therefore, these devices now are available in the United States for investigational use only.[28] Patients who meet the criteria for the approved HDE indication (treatment of patients who have recurrent cryptogenic stroke caused by presumed paradoxical embolism through a PFO and who have not responded to conventional drug therapy) have access to these devices through an Investigational Device Exemption.[31] In addition to PFO and secundum atrial septal defect closure, these devices have been used to close muscular and perimembranous ventricular septal defects (either congenital or acquired).[32–34] Closure of a perimembranous or a muscular ventricular defect has been reported to be successful approximately 96% of the time, with a major complication rate of 2%.[34] Success rates for closure of PFOs and atrial septal defects have ranged from 79% to 100% after several years' follow-up.[23]

Complications related to the deployment of septal occluder devices require immediate recognition, evaluation, and treatment to prevent permanent sequelae or minimize their impact.[35] Complications include, but are not limited to, intraprocedure air embolism; device embolization; device positioning; device thrombosis and embolization (cerebral embolization may occur from air, a piece of the device itself, or thrombus) during or following the procedure; device-related arrhythmias (usually atrial, but sudden death has occurred); and cardiac perforation with or without cardiac tamponade.[28,35] These devices are placed in the cardiac catheterization laboratory with the aid of fluoroscopy and ultrasound guidance. Cardiac ultrasound may either be performed with TEE or intracardiac echocardiography. TEE requires endotracheal intubation and general anesthesia, because the patient must remain still to allow precise placement of the occluder devices. Intracardiac ultrasound does not require endotracheal intubation or general anesthesia but still demands the presence of a cardiac anesthesiologist. The anesthesiologist/cardiologist team ensures optimal patient comfort and allows the cardiologist to devote attention wholly to performing the procedure while remaining vigilant for any complication that may arise.

Peripheral Arterial Disease

Approximately 8 million Americans are afflicted with lower-extremity peripheral arterial disease.[36] This disease is a result of atherosclerotic occlusion of the peripheral arteries and increases in prevalence after 40 years of age.[37] As in coronary artery disease, the prevalence is slightly higher in men than in women.[38] The principle symptom of occlusive peripheral arterial disease is intermittent claudication. (The term "claudication" is derived from the Latin term "claudicaro," meaning "to limp").[39] Because of insufficient arterial blood flow and leg ischemia, patients who suffer from intermittent claudication may have symptoms of pain, aching, a sense of fatigue, or other discomfort that is experienced in the affected muscle group with exercise, especially walking, and is relieved with rest.[39] Symptoms usually are located in the muscle bed supplied by the most proximal stenosis.[39] Obstruction of the aorta or iliac flow typically results in buttock, hip, or thigh claudication. Femoral or popliteal arterial stenosis commonly results in calf claudication, and ankle or pedal claudication occurs as a result of either tibial or peroneal disease.[39]

The American College of Cardiology/American Heart Association and other guidelines suggest that percutaneous revascularization be considered in patients who have intermittent claudication when[40–42]

Exercise rehabilitation and pharmacologic therapy have not been successful in providing the patient with an adequate response

Claudication symptoms significantly disable the patient, resulting in an inability to perform normal work or other important activities

The procedure carries a very favorable risk/benefit ratio and has a high likelihood of initial and long-term success

The patient is able to benefit from an improvement in claudication (ie, exercise is not limited by another cause, such as angina, heart failure, chronic obstructive pulmonary disease, or orthopedic problems)

The characteristics of the lesion permit appropriate intervention at low risk with a high likelihood of initial and long-term success

The patient has limb-threatening ischemia, as manifested by rest pain, ischemic ulcers, or gangrene

In lower-extremity stent procedures, epidural anesthesia may attenuate stress responses and reduce the production of acute-phase reactants, leading to fewer complications related to hypercoagulation.[43] A major concern regarding regional blocks is the risk for an epidural or a spinal hematoma, because most of these patients are taking antithrombotic medications (eg, clopidogrel, aspirin, warfarin, or heparin).[44,45] The anesthesiologist may be of great benefit to the interventional cardiologist during a peripheral vascular intervention. Many of these patients have resting claudication that precludes them from lying still during the procedure. In addition, performance of endovascular intervention, with or without stent implantation, frequently is associated with transient painful leg ischemia that may lead to patient movement and further increase the risk of complication.

Percutaneous Valve Repair and Replacement

Although percutaneous valvuloplasty for mitral, aortic, and pulmonic stenosis has been performed for decades, newer percutaneous techniques for the treatment of mitral regurgitation and percutaneous aortic valve replacement have been developed only recently and are presently under investigation.[46–48]

Percutaneous mitral valve repair

Cardiac surgical mitral valve repair is currently the procedure of choice for the treatment of symptomatic mitral regurgitation or mitral regurgitation with impaired left ventricular ejection fraction (< 60%). Current techniques for percutaneous mitral valve repair include coronary sinus annuloplasty, direct annuloplasty, leaflet repair, and chamber plus annular remodeling.[49]

Because the coronary sinus runs parallel to the mitral annulus, a device can be placed within the sinus to deform the annulus and decrease the annular circumference.[49] One device uses anchors or stents percutaneously placed in the coronary sinus ostium and the distal coronary sinus. These anchors are bridged by a connecting spring (the Monarc device, Edwards Lifesciences Inc., Orange, California). Tension develops as the spring shortens and the coronary sinus diminishes in diameter. The Carillon mitral contour system (Cardiac Dimensions, Kirkland, Washington) is another percutaneous coronary device system that uses a nitinol wire-shaping ribbon between the proximal and distal anchors.[50–52] The efficacy of these devices is being evaluated.

In many patients the coronary sinus does not directly parallel the mitral annulus, and in about half of the patients the coronary sinus crosses over branches of the circumflex coronary artery.[53] Compression of the circumflex coronary artery may occur at the time of implantation or, in the case of the Monarc device, later as the biodegradable material in the spring spaces absorbs and the spring element shortens over a period of weeks to months.[49] Other complications of coronary sinus–based procedures may include coronary sinus erosion or thrombosis. Therefore, the safety and the efficacy of the coronary sinus approach remains to be determined.

In the early 1990s Alfieri[54,55] demonstrated that suturing the free mitral valve leaflet edges of the midpart of the line of mitral coaptation creates a mitral valve with a double orifice. Although isolated edge-to-edge mitral valve repair may be durable in selected patients with 5-year 90% freedom from re-operation and mitral regurgitation more than 2 + or moderate mitral regurgitation,[56] this technique also has had mixed clinical results.[57,58]

The MitraClip (Evalve, San Francisco, California) is a percutaneously delivered device that duplicates the Alfieri edge-to-edge repair. After a transatrial septal puncture is made, the clip is positioned in the mid-left atrium cavity above the mitral valve orifice. The clip is positioned in the center of the valve orifice and is aligned above the origin of the mitral regurgitant jet. The clip then is opened and passed into the left ventricular cavity and is drawn back so that the mitral valve leaflets are grasped. Once the leaflets are grasped, the clip is closed to create a double-orifice mitral valve.[59,60] In a phase I clinical trial, the rate of 2-year freedom from death, mitral valve surgery, or recurrent mitral regurgitation > 2 + was 80% in patients undergoing successful clip therapy.[61] The success of the Evalve clip procedure in this phase I trial has led to a randomized trial comparing this procedure with mitral valve surgery in selected patients, the Endovascular Valve Edge to Edge Repair Study II trial.[49]

Presently, all patients undergoing percutaneous mitral valve repair using the Evalve procedure receive general anesthesia. Placement of the device is guided by fluoroscopy and TEE.[23]

Percutaneous aortic valve replacement

Cribier[47] developed the first percutaneous heart valve for humans based on the initial animal work of Anderson and Pavcnik and colleagues.[62] Presently, percutaneous aortic valve replacement is performed in patients who have severe aortic stenosis, New York Heart Association class IV symptoms related to aortic stenosis, and comorbidities that exclude them from cardiac surgery because of excessive risk.[63] Ongoing randomized, controlled clinical trials are comparing surgical aortic valve replacement and percutaneous aortic valve replacement using newer-generation percutaneous aortic prosthetic valves in patients who are candidates for cardiac surgery.[64] Some experts in this field believe that, depending on the trial results and future technological advances, percutaneous aortic valve replacement may be a viable option for a patient in need of a prosthetic aortic valve to avoid the concomitant complications inherent in open heart surgery.[64]

The Cribier-Edwards aortic valve (Edwards Lifesciences, Irvine, California) consists of three bovine pericardial leaflets sutured to a stainless steel balloon expandable stent. The valve is crimped on an aortic valvuloplasty balloon that is expandable to 23 to 26 mm (NuMED Inc., Hopkinton, New York). This system is delivered through a 24-F (8-mm) sheath with an antegrade approach using a transatrial septal puncture. Once the sheath is positioned across the native aortic valve, the prosthetic aortic valve is delivered and placed in the aortic position through rapid inflation and deflation of the balloon. Antegrade flow is minimized temporarily by high-rate pacing.[63] Cribier[65] recently reported a series of 35 patients undergoing this procedure. Twenty-seven of the 35 patients underwent a successful implantation with improvement of aortic valve area and left ventricular function. Five patients developed moderately severe aortic insufficiency. There were no device-related deaths in 9 to 26 months of follow-up.[65] More recently an antegrade approach has been developed that is not as technically demanding and may be safer.[66]

Currently, technological advances are occurring in the development of percutaneous delivered aortic valves. The CoreValve (CoreValve, Inc., Paris, France) is a percutaneous aortic valve that is self expanding and consists of a bioprosthetic pericardial tissue valve sutured in a nitinol metal stent.[63] Preliminary studies have demonstrated that an advantage of this self-expanding stent-valve system is lack of significant aortic regurgitation.[63] Other percutaneously delivered aortic valves are being developed (eg, by AorTx, Inc., Redwood City, California) that may be retrieved after deployment. It is believed that these advances in technology will lead to valves that are more deliverable and safer.[63]

On September 5, 2007 Edwards Lifesciences Corporation announced European approval for commercial release of the Edwards SAPIEN transcatheter aortic valve technology with the RetroFlex transfemoral delivery system.[67] This bovine pericardial tissue valve is constructed with a cobalt chromium alloy stent that reduces the profile of the system by 4 to 5 F as compared with the other systems described previously. The reduced diameter of this delivery system allows easier access into and within the patient's vasculature through a smaller catheter and may lead to a lower risk of procedural complication.[68] This valve presently is being studies in the Placement of Aortic Transcatheter Valve trial in high-risk symptomatic patients who have severe aortic stenosis.[68] This valve also may be placed in the aorta via a transapical approach with the Ascendra delivery system.[68]

The initial clinical experience with the transapical transcatheter approach for aortic valve implantation in humans was reported in 2006.[69] This approach uses a left anterolateral intercostals incision to expose the left ventricular apex. A hemostatic sheath is introduced by direct needle puncture of the apex. The prosthetic valve is crimped onto a valvuloplasty balloon and is passed over a wire into the left ventricular cavity. Fluoroscopy, aortography, and echocardiography confirm proper positioning. As in the percutaneous technique, rapid ventricular pacing is used to decrease cardiac output while the balloon is inflated and the prosthesis is deployed within the annulus. The initial experience was reported on seven patients. There were no procedural deaths. One death occurred in the 7 patients during a mean follow-up of 87 ± 56 days.[69] Since the first report, other published reports have demonstrated safety with good early results in high-risk patients.[70,71]

Cardiac anesthesiologists are needed for the performance of percutaneous aortic valve replacement. These patients are extremely ill and frequently need endotracheal intubation and general anesthesia. In addition, they often are hemodynamically unstable and are at high risk for cardiac death during the procedure.

ELECTROPHYSIOLOGY INTERVENTIONS

The current era of clinical electrophysiology that began in 1960s has evolved from simple diagnostic procedures to therapeutic interventions. In recent years, the number of electrophysiology procedures has increased exponentially.

The complexity and length of these procedures also have evolved dramatically and frequently mandate administration of different analgesics and moderate sedation. Although electrophysiologists commonly administer a combination of narcotics and benzodiazepine for conscious sedation, consultation with a cardiac anesthesiologist frequently is required to manage and stabilize a spectrum of patient profiles ranging from healthy young patients who have no significant cardiac history or comorbidities to patients who have advanced heart failure and multisystem disease. Therefore, the anesthesiologist's understanding of electrophysiology procedures is key in determining the outcome. This section reviews current electrophysiology procedures.

Electrophysiology Studies

Electrophysiology studies are performed to evaluate specific arrhythmias, specific symptoms, or events such as syncope, palpitation, or cardiac arrest that suggest the occurrence of an arrhythmia.[72] Catheters commonly are placed via femoral venous access into the high right atrium, His bundle, coronary sinus, right ventricular apex, or right ventricular outflow tract. Programmed stimulation is performed from the high right atrium, right ventricular apex, or right ventricular outflow tract to induce ventricular or supraventricular tachycardias as well as to help identify etiologies of bradyarrhythmias. These procedures usually are performed with conscious sedation and light analgesics. Drugs that may affect the sympathetic and parasympathetic nervous systems should be avoided, because they commonly influence the function of the atrioventricular node and sinus node and thus may affect inducibility of certain arrhythmias.

Catheter Ablation

Catheter ablation is commonly used to treat supraventricular tachyarrhythmias such as atrioventricular nodal re-entry tachycardia, tachycardias related to Wolf-Parkinson-White syndrome, and atrial flutter. More recently, catheter ablation also has been used to treat atrial fibrillation. Radiofrequency is the energy most commonly used.[73] Radiofrequency catheter ablation has been used as a first-line treatment for some arrhythmias as well as a treatment for arrhythmias that are refractory to pharmacologic therapy.[72] The major arrhythmias that have been treated with radiofrequency ablation include: A-V nodal re-entrant tachycardia; atrial ventricular re-entrant tachycardia associated with the Wolf-Parkinson-White syndrome and an atrial ventricular bypass tract; atrial flutter; bundle branch re-entry ventricular tachycardia; and atrial fibrillation.

Radiofrequency ablation also has been used as an adjunctive therapy for recurrent ventricular tachycardia caused by coronary artery disease or arrhythmogenic right ventricular dysplasia.[73] As in an electrophysiology study, in catheter ablation procedures catheters are placed in different cardiac chambers, and programmed stimulation is performed from different sites to induce tachyarrhythmias. In addition, different medications (isoproterenol, epinephrine, dopamine, aminophylline, atropine, adenosine, beta-blockers, ibutilide, verapamil, procainamide, and others) are used to induce and terminate tachyarrhythmias.[72]

Radiofrequency ablation procedures require complex mapping techniques to identify the source of the arrhythmia and specify the exact location of radiofrequency ablation. These mapping techniques include activation mapping; pace mapping; entrainment mapping; anatomic fluoroscopy-based, three-dimensional (3D) electroanatomic mapping; 3D noncontact mapping, and intracardiac echo-guided anatomic mapping. All these techniques and the application of radiofrequency ablation energy require that patient lie still on the electrophysiology table for the accurate localization of the arrhythmogenic focus. Patient comfort often becomes an issue, and deeper sedation is necessary. Therefore the role of the anesthesiologist becomes crucial in facilitating ablation procedures by maintaining a patient's airway and ensuring hemodynamic stability with minimal movement of the patient's body.

Once an arrhythmia is diagnosed and localized, energy sources other than radiofrequency may be applied to destroy the arrhythmogenic focus. These energy sources include cryothermic energy, ultrasound, laser, and microwave. Regardless of the energy source delivered to specific targets, the patient may experience pain and may require more sedation.

Radiofrequency ablation procedures are becoming more tedious and time consuming. Patients who have atrial fibrillation may require a procedure time of 6 to 8 hours, followed by a 30-minute observation time after ablation and repeat electrophysiology testing to ensure success of the procedure.[72]

Electrical Cardioversion

Electrical cardioversion ideally requires an anesthesiologist. Cardiologists frequently have administered conscious sedation with benzodiazepines alone, with suboptimal results.[74] The authors recommend that all patients who undergo elective electrical cardioversion receive conscious sedation under the direction of an anesthesiologist to minimize patient discomfort and promote rapid recovery.

Implantable Cardioverter Defibrillators

Large, prospective, multicenter, randomized trials in patients who had coronary and noncoronary heart disease and a wide range of ventricular function have demonstrated the efficacy and safety of implantable cardioverter defibrillators (ICDs).[75] Indications for ICD implantation include both the primary and secondary prevention of ventricular tachycardia and/or ventricular fibrillation to decrease the risk of sudden cardiac death.[75] With the advent of smaller biphasic transvenous ICDs and the experience gained over the years, it now is feasible for electrophysiologists to implant ICDs safely in the pectoral area without surgical assistance. Throughout the years, general anesthesia has been the standard anesthesia technique used for these procedures, but the use of local anesthesia combined with conscious sedation has facilitated and simplified these procedures further. It is feasible to use local anesthesia for current ICD implants to expedite the procedure and avoid the cost and possible complications related to general anesthesia. The role of anesthesiologist is crucial during defibrillation threshold testing, when deeper sedation or occasionally general anesthesia is required in patients who generally have significant comorbidities and significant left ventricular dysfunction.

Defibrillation threshold testing can be considered the most critical part of the ICD implantation procedure. Although the risk associated with defibrillation threshold testing usually is low, serious complications may occur as a consequence of this practice. These complications include transient ischemic attack, stroke, cardiopulmonary arrest caused by refractory ventricular fibrillation, pulseless electrical activity, cardiogenic shock, embolic events, and death.[76,77] In unstable patients or patients who have untreated coronary artery disease, defibrillation threshold testing usually is omitted because of the potential life-threatening risks of the procedure.

Biventricular Pacing and Defibrillation Lead Placement

Cardiac resynchronization therapy with defibrillation systems is prescribed for both primary and secondary prevention of sudden cardiac death in patients who have heart failure associated with an ischemic or a non-ischemic origin. The presently recommended criteria for implantation of a biventricular pacemaker with defibrillation capability includes patients who have a left ventricular ejection fraction of less than 35% with a wide (> 120 ms) QRS complex and drug-refractory New York Heart Association class III or IV heart failure who are receiving optimal medical therapy for their heart failure.[76–78]

These patients may be unable to lie flat on the electrophysiology table because of their advanced heart failure and increased total lung water despite diuretic therapy. Therefore, close monitoring of the patient's blood pressure, heart rate, and oxygenation is extremely important. The skill of an anesthesiologist is required to administer conscious sedation gradually to avoid cardiac decompensation during these generally long procedures. Positioning the left ventricular lead via the coronary sinus and great cardiac vein can be a very complex and lengthy procedure because of distorted ventricular anatomy. Generally these patients have severe right ventricular and left ventricular dilatation and valvular regurgitation that may complicate lead positioning. Lead dislodgement may occur immediately after lead placement, further prolonging these procedures.

Procedure-related complications can include the development of refractory heart failure. Therefore, the need for airway protection is critical, and the ability to intubate the patient is crucial to the success of the procedure and survival of the patient. Other complications can include pneumothorax and coronary sinus perforation related to lead placement. Coronary sinus perforation may be recognized clinically by contrast extravasation. Cardiac tamponade may occur as a result of perforation of the coronary sinus or from cardiac perforation related to ventricular or atrial lead placement. The development of cardiac tamponade necessitates immediate pericardiocentesis upon recognition.

TRANSESOPHAGEAL ECHOCARDIOGRAPHY

The clinical indications for TEE continue to be defined. In two large series, the clinical indications for TEE were for cardiac sources of embolism (36%), endocarditis (14%), prosthetic heart valve function (12%), native valvular disease, aortic dissection or aneurysm, intracardiac tumor, mass, or thrombus (6%–8% each), and congenital heart disease (4%).[79,80] In current practice, TEE commonly is performed with most major cardiac surgical procedures to verify preoperative diagnoses, monitor ventricular function, and assess the success of valve repair.[81] The 2007 appropriateness criteria from the American Society of Echocardiography include the following indications for TEE as an initial test:[82]

Evaluation of suspected aortic dissection
Guidance during percutaneous interventions for structural heart disease
Determining suitability for valve repair
Diagnosis of endocarditis
Evaluation of persistent fever with an intracardiac device
Evaluation for left atrial thrombus or spontaneous echo contrast before cardioversion or radiofrequency ablation

As compared with transthoracic echocardiography, TEE offers superior visualization of posterior cardiac structures because of the close proximity of the esophagus to the posteromedial heart with the absence of intervening lung and bone. This proximity permits the use of high-frequency imaging transducers that afford superior spatial resolution.[83] TEE is contraindicated in the presence of the following conditions: esophageal stricture or malignancy; surgical interposition of the esophagus; recent esophageal ulcer or hemorrhage; Zenker's diverticulum; altered mental status or an uncooperative patient; and a history of odynophagia or dysphagia in the absence of a screening endoscopy and or barium swallow.[83]

Risk of bleeding increases in patients who are taking anticoagulants, who have received thrombolytic therapy before the procedure, who are thrombocytopenic, or who have other bleeding disorders. The risk of bleeding in patients who have esophageal varices is not known but probably is increased.[83]

Description of Procedure and the Role of Anesthesia

Although considered moderately invasive, the performance of a TEE requires the focused attention of the cardiologist and is performed best in combination with an anesthesiologist. In patients who are difficult to intubate with the TEE probe, the anesthesiologist can visualize the glottis directly with a laryngoscope and facilitate an uncomplicated successful esophageal intubation. In uncooperative patients, a greater level of sedation and prophylactic tracheal intubation for airway protection also can be helpful.

Careful attention to topical posterior pharyngeal anesthesia with Cetacaine spray (Cetylite Industries, Inc., Pennsauken, New Jersey) and patient reassurance ("verbal anesthesia") helps minimize the degree of sedation that is required. Pulse oximetry is used to monitor oxygen saturation. Intravenous glycopyrrolate can be administered to decrease secretions during the procedure. Because of its anticholinergic properties, glycopyrrolate inhibits salivation and excessive pharyngeal secretions, reducing the risk of aspiration pneumonia.

Serious complications of TEE, including death, sustained ventricular tachycardia, and severe angina, have been estimated at less than 1 in 5000.[79,80] There is a low risk of pharyngeal, esophageal, or stomach perforation. In a study of 10,000 consecutive patients undergoing TEE, there was one case of hypopharyngeal perforation, two cases of cervical esophageal perforation, and no fatalities.[84]

Application of topical benzocaine and related agents that are used for posterior pharyngeal anesthesia may be associated with the development of methemoglobinemia, a potentially life-threatening complication. The development of cyanosis in the presence of normal arterial oxygen saturation is an indication of the development of methemoglobinemia.[85,86] Therefore, pulse oximetry cannot be used to make a diagnosis of methemoglobinemia. Minor complications include transient bronchospasm, transient hypoxia, nonsustained ventricular tachycardia, transient atrial fibrillation, vomiting, pharyngeal abrasion, and pharyngeal hematoma.[83]

SUMMARY

As described throughout this article, modern invasive cardiovascular procedures are complex and demand the full attention of the attending cardiologist and the complete cooperation of the patient. In many, if not most, of the circumstances described here, the anesthesiologist is a welcome addition to the cardiovascular team. The anesthesiologist's knowledge, skills, abilities, and experience are invaluable in ensuring optimal procedure results and good patient outcomes.

REFERENCES

1. North American Society of Pacing and Electrophysiology consensus statement on the use of conscious sedation. Pacing Clin Electrophysiol 1998;21(2):375–85.
2. Popma JJ. Coronary arteriography and intravascular imaging. In: Libby P, Bonow R, editors. Braunwald's heart disease: a textbook of cardiovascular medicine. 8th edition. Philadelphia: Saunders Elsevier; 2007. p. 465–508.
3. Davidson CJ, Bonow RO. Cardiac catheterization. In: Libby P, Bonow R, editors. Braunwald's heart disease: a textbook of cardiovascular medicine. 8th edition. [chapter 19]. Philadelphia: Saunders Elsevier; 2007. p. 439.
4. Scanlon PJ, Faxon DP, Audet AM, et al. ACC/AHA guidelines for coronary arteriography: executive summary and recommendations. A report of the American College of Cardiology/American Heart Association Task Force On Practice Guidelines (committee on coronary angiography) Developed in Collaboration with the Society for Cardiac Angiography and Interventions. Circulation 1999;99:2345–57.
5. Mintz GS, Popma JJ, Pichard AD, et al. Limitations of angiography in the assessment of plaque distribution in coronary artery disease: a systematic study of target lesion eccentricity in 1446 lesions. Circulation 1996;93(5):924–31.
6. Bayshore TM, Bates ER, Berger PB, et al. ACC/SCAI clinical expert consensus document on cardiac catheterization laboratory standards. J Am Coll Cardiol 2001;37:2170.
7. Smith SC Jr, Feldman TE, Hirshfeld JW Jr, et al. ACC/AHA/SCAI 2005 guideline update for percutaneous coronary intervention: a report of the American college of cardiology/american heart association task force on practice guidelines (ACC/AHA/SCAI writing committee to update the 2001 guidelines for percutaneous coronary intervention). J Am Coll Cardiol 2006;47(1):e7.
8. Thygesen K, Alpert JS, White HD. On behalf of the joint ESC/ACCF/AHA/WHF Task Force for the Redefinition of Myocardial Infarction. Universal definition of myocardial infarction. Eur Heart J 2007;28(20):2525–38.

9. The TIMI IIIB Investigators. Effects of tissue plasminogen activator and a comparison of early invasive and conservative strategies in unstable angina and non-Q-wave myocardial infarction. Results of the TIMI IIIB trial. Thrombolysis in Myocardial Ischemia. Circulation 1994;89(4):1545–56.

10. Anderson HV, Cannon CP, Stone PH, et al. One-year results of the thrombolysis in myocardial infarction (TIMI) IIIB clinical trial. A randomized comparison of tissue-type plasminogen activator versus placebo and early invasive versus early conservative strategies in unstable angina and non-Q wave myocardial infarction. J Am Coll Cardiol 1995;26(7):1643–50.

11. Boden WE, O'Rourke RA, Teo KK, et al. Optimal medical therapy with or without PCI for stable coronary artery disease. N Engl J Med 2007;356:1503–16.

12. Huang HW, Brent B, Shaw R. Trends in percutaneous versus surgical revascularization of unprotected left main coronary stenosis in the drug-eluting stent era— a report from the American college of cardiology national cardiovascular data registry. Catheter Cardiovasc Interv 2006;68:867–72.

13. Jones RH. Percutaneous intervention vs. coronary artery bypass grafting in left main coronary artery disease [editorial]. N Engl J Med 2008;358:1851.

14. Biondi-Zoccai GGI, Lotrionte M, Morett C, et al. A collaborative systematic review and meta-analysis on 1278 patients undergoing percutaneous drug-eluting stenting for unprotected left main coronary artery disease. Am Heart J 2008;155: 274–83.

15. Seung KB, Park DW, Young-Hak K, et al. Stents versus coronary-artery bypass grafting for left main coronary artery disease. N Engl J Med 2008;358(17): 1781–93.

16. Motwani JG, Raymond RE, Franco I, et al. Effectiveness of rotational atherectomy of right coronary artery ostial stenosis. Am J Cardiol 2000;85:563.

17. MacIsaac AI, Bass TA, Buchbinder M, et al. High speed rotational atherectomy; outcome in calcified and noncalcified coronary artery lesions. J Am Coll Cardiol 1995;26:73.

18. Pretorius M, Hughes AK, Stahlman MB, et al. Placement of the tandemheart percutaneous left ventricular assist device. Anesthesiology 2006;103:1412–3.

19. Kar B, Adkins LE, Civitello AB, et al. Clinical experience with the TandemHeart percutaneous ventricular assist device. Tex Heart Inst J 2006;33:111–5.

20. Henriques JP, Remmelink M, Baan J Jr, et al. Safety and feasibility of elective high-risk percutaneous coronary intervention procedures with left ventricular support of the Impella Recover LP 2.5. Am J Cardiol 2006;97: 990–2.

21. Siegenthaler MP, Brehm K, Strecher T, et al. The Impella recover microaxial left ventricular assist device reduces mortality for postcardiotomy failure: a three-center experience. J Thorac Cardiovasc Surg 2004;127:812–22.

22. Windecker S, Meier B. Impella assisted high-risk percutaneous coronary intervention. Karddiovask Med 2005;8:187–9.

23. Shook DC, Gross W. Offsite anesthesiology in the cardiac catheterization lab. Curr Opin Anaesthesiol 2007;20:352–8.

24. FDA. Available at: http://www/fda.gov/cdrh/mda/docs/p000039.html. Accessed June 2008.

25. Bayard YL, Ostermayer SH, Hein R, et al. Percutaneous devices for stroke prevention. Cardiovasc Revasc Med 2007;8:216–25.

26. Pinto Slottow TL, Steinberg DH, Waksman R. Overview of the 2007 food and drug administration circulatory system devices panel meeting on patent foramen ovale closure devices. Circulation 2007;116:677–82.

27. Amplazer Septal Occluder. AGA Medical Corporation. Available at: http://www.amplatzer.com/products/asd_devices/tabid/179/default.aspx. Accessed February 25, 2009.
28. Wiegers SE, St. John Sutton MG. Devices for percutaneous closure of a secundum atrial septal defect. Available at: www.uptodate.com. Accessed June 2008.
29. Pedra CA, Pihkla J, Lee KJ, et al. Transcatheter closure of atrial septal defects using the CardioSeal implant. Heart 2000;84:320.
30. Carminati M, Chessa M, Butera G, et al. Transcatheter closure of atrial septal defects with the STARFlex device: early results and follow up. J Interv Cardiol 2001; 14:319.
31. FDA. Available at: http://www.fda.gov/cdrh/ode/h000007-h990011withdrawl.html. Accessed June 2008.
32. Wiegers SE, St. John Sutton MG. Management of atrial septal defects in adults. Available at: www.uptodate.com. Accessed June 2008.
33. Valente AM, Rhodes JF. Current indications and contraindications for transcatheter atrial septal defect and patent foramen ovale device closure. Am Heart J 2007;153(4):81–4.
34. Butera G, Chessa M, Carminati M. Percutaneous closure of ventricular septal defects. Cardiol Young 2007;17:243–53.
35. Carroll JD, Dodge S, Groves BM. Percutaneous patent foramen ovale closure. Cardiol Clin 2005;23:13–33.
36. Thom T, Hasse N, Rosamond W, et al. Heart disease and stroke statistics—2006 update: a report from the American Heart Association Statistics Committee and Stroke Statistics Subcommittee. Circulation 2006;113:e85.
37. Selvin E, Erlinger TP. Prevalence of and risk factors for peripheral arterial disease in the United States: results from the national health and nutrition examination survey, 1999–2000. Circulation 2004;110:738.
38. Hirsch AT, Haskal ZJ, Hertzer NR, et al. ACC/AHA 2005 guidelines for the management of patients with peripheral arterial disease (lower extremity, renal, mesenteric, and abdominal aortic): a collaborative report from the American Association for Vascular Surgery/Society for Vascular Surgery, Society for Cardiovascular Angiography and Interventions, Society for Vascular Medicine and Biology, Society of Interventional Radiology, and the ACC/AHA Task Force on Practice Guidelines (Writing Committee to Develop Guidelines for the Management of Patients with Peripheral Arterial Disease). Available at: http://www.acc.org/clinical/guidelines/pad/index.pdf. Accessed February 25, 2009.
39. Creager MA, Libby P. Peripheral arterial diseases. In: Libby P, Bonow R, editors. Braunwald's heart disease: a textbook of cardiovascular medicine. 8th edition. Philadelphia: Saunders Elsevier; 2007.
40. Hirsch AT, Haskal ZJ, Hertzer NR, et al. ACC/AHA 2005 practice guidelines for the management of patients with peripheral arterial disease (lower extremity, renal, mesenteric, and abdominal aortic): a collaborative report from the American Association for Vascular Surgery/Society for Vascular Surgery, Society for Cardiovascular Angiography and Interventions, Society for Vascular Medicine and Biology, Society of Interventional Radiology, and the ACC/AHA Task Force on Practice Guidelines (Writing Committee to Develop Guidelines for the Management of Patients with Peripheral Arterial Disease): Endorsed by the American Association of Cardiovascular and Pulmonary Rehabilitation; National Heart, Lung, And Blood Institute; Society for Vascular Nursing; Transatlantic Inter-Society Consensus; and Vascular Disease Foundation. Circulation 2006;113: e463.

41. Norgen L, Hiatt WR, Dormandy JA, et al. Inter-society consensus for the management of peripheral arterial disease (TASC II). J Vasc Surg 2007;45(Suppl S):S5.
42. Pell JP. Impact of intermittent claudication on quality of life. The Scottish Vascular Audit Group. Eur J Vasc Endovasc Surg 1995;9:469.
43. Tuman KJ, McCarthy RJ, March RJ, et al. Effects of epidural anesthesia and analgesia on coagulation and outcome after major vascular surgery. Anesthesiology 1991;73(6):696–704.
44. Vandermeulen EP, Van Aken H, Vermylen J. Anticoagulants and spinal-epidural anesthesia. Anesth Analg 1994;79:1165–77, 17.
45. Onishchuk JL, Carlsson C. Epidural hematoma associated with epidural anesthesia: complications of anticoagulant therapy. Anesthesiology 1992;77: 1221–3.
46. Vassiliades TA, Block PC, Cohn LH, et al. The clinical development of percutaneous heart valve technology: a position statement of the society of thoracic surgeons, the American Association for Thoracic Surgery and the Society for Cardiovascular Angiography and Interventions Endorsed by the American College of Cardiology Foundation and the American Heart Association. J Am Coll Cardiol 2005;45:1554–60.
47. Cribier A, Eltchaninoff H, Bash A, et al. Percutaneous transcatheter implantation of an aortic valve prostheses for calcific aortic stenosis: first human case description. Circulation 2002;106:3006–8.
48. Cribier A, Eltchaninoff H, Tron C, et al. Percutaneous implantation of aortic valve prosthesis in patients with calcific aortic stenosis: technical advances, clinical results and future strategies. J Interv Cardiol 2006;19:S87–96.
49. Feldman T. Percutaneous mitral valve repair. J Interv Cardiol 2007;20(6):488–94.
50. Byrne MJ, Power JM, Alferness CA, et al. Percutaneous mitral annular reduction. A novel approach to the management of heart failure associated mitral regurgitation. Circulation 2003;108:1795–9.
51. Maniu CV, Patel JB, Reuter DG, et al. Percutaneous mitral annular reduction provides continued benefit in an ovine model of dilated cardiomyopathy. Circulation 2004;110:3088–92.
52. Liddicoat JR, MacNeill BD, Gillinov AM, et al. Percutaneous mitral valve repair: a feasibility study in an ovine model of acute ischemic mitral regurgitation. Catheter Cardiovasc Interv 2003;60:410–6.
53. Maselli D, Guarracino F, Chiaramonti F, et al. Percutaneous mitral annuloplasty: an anatomic study of human coronary sinus and its relation with mitral valve annulus and coronary arteries. Circulation 2006;114:377–80.
54. Alfieri O, Maisano F, DeBonis M, et al. The edge-to-edge technique in mitral valve repair: a simple solution for complex problems. J Thorac Cardiovasc Surg 2001; 122:674–81.
55. Alfieri O, Elefteriades JA, Chapolini RJ, et al. Novel suture device for beating-heart mitral leaflet approximation. Ann Thorac Surg 2002;74:1488–93.
56. Maaisano F, Vigano G, Blasio A, et al. Surgical isolated edge-to-edge mitral repair without annuloplasty—clinical proof of principle for an endovascular approach. Eurointerv 2006;2:181–6.
57. Bhudia SK, McCarthy PM, Smedira NG, et al. Edge-to-edge (Alfieri) mitral repair: results in diverse clinical settings. Ann Thorac Surg 2004;77:1598–606.
58. Kherani AR, Cheema FH, Casher J, et al. Edge-to-edge mitral valve repair: the Columbia Presbyterian experience. Ann Thorac Surg 2004;78:73–6.
59. St. Goar FG, James FI, Komtebedde J, et al. Endovascular edge-to-edge mitral valve repair: short-term results in a porcine model. Circulation 2003;108:1990–3.

60. Fann JI, St. Goar FG, Komtebedde J, et al. Off-pump edge-to-edge mitral valve technique using a mechanical clip in a chronic model. Circulation 2003; 108(Suppl IV):493.
61. Feldman T, Wasserman H, Herrmann HC, et al. Edge-to-edge mitral valve repair using the Evalve MitraClip: one year results of the EVEREST phase I clinical trial. Am J Cardiol 2005;96(Suppl):49H.
62. Pavcnik D, Wright KC, Wallace S. Development and initial experimental evaluation of a prosthetic aortic valve for transcatheter placement. Work in progress. Radiology 1992;183:151–4.
63. Rajagopal V, Kapadia SR, Tuzcu EM. Advances in the percutaneous treatment of aortic and mitral valve disease. Minerva Cardioangiol 2007;55:83–94.
64. Webb JG. New treatment options in aortic stenosis. American College of Cardiology Extended Learning Program 2008;40(4), disc 1.
65. Cribier A, Eltchaninoff H, Tron C, et al. Treatment of calcific aortic stenosis with the percutaneous heart valve: mid-term follow-up from the initial feasibility studies: the French experience. J Am Coll Cardiol 2006;47:1214–23.
66. Webb JG, Chandavimol M, Thompson DR, et al. Percutaneous aortic valve implantation retrograde from the femoral artery. Circulation 2006;113:842–50.
67. Edwards Lifesciences Corporation. Available at: http://www.edwards.com/newsroom/nr20070905.htm. Accessed February 25, 2009.
68. Edwards Lifesciences Corporation. Available at: http://medgadget.com/archives/2008/03/edwards_sapien_transcatheter_aortic_valve_makes_human_debut.html. Accessed February 25, 2009.
69. Lichtesnstein SV, Cheung A, Ye J, et al. Transapical transcatheter aortic valve implantation in humans: initial clinical experience. Circulation 2006;114:591–6.
70. Walther T, Simon P, Dewey T, et al. Transapical minimally invasive aortic valve implantation multicenter experience. Circulation 2007;116(Suppl 1):240–5.
71. Walther T, Falk V, Borger MA, et al. Minimally invasive transapical beating heart aortic valve implantation – proof of concept. Eur J Cardiothorac Surg 2007;31: 9–15.
72. ACC/AHA/HRS Writing Committee. ACC/AHA/HRS 2006 key data elements and definitions for electrophysiological studies and procedures: a report of the American College of Cardiology/American Heart Association Task Force on Clinical Data Standards (Acc/Aha/Hrs Writing Committee to Develop Data Standards on Electrophysiology). Circulation 2006;114:2534–70 [originally published online Nov 27, 2006].
73. Ganz L. Catheter ablation of cardiac arrhythmias: overview and technical aspects. Available at: www.uptodate.com. Accessed June 2008.
74. Kudoh A, Takase H, Takahira Y, et al. Postoperative confusion increases in elderly long-term benzodiazepine users. Anesthesiology 2004;99(6):1674–8.
75. Gregoratos G, Abrahms J, Epstein A, et al. ACC/AHA/NASPE 2002 guideline update for implantation of cardiac pacemakers and antiarrhythmia devices: summary article: a report of the American College of Cardiology/American Heart Association Task Force on Practice Guidelines. Circulation 2002;106: 2145–61.
76. Brignole M, Raciti G, Bongiorni MG, et al. Testing at the time of implantation of cardioverter defibrillator in clinical practice: a nation-wide survey. Europace 2007;9(7):540–3.
77. McAlister FA, Ezekowitz JA, Wiebe N, et al. Systematic review: cardiac resynchronization in patients with symptomatic heart failure. Ann Intern Med 2004;141: 381–90.

78. Boriani G, Biffi M, Martignani C, et al. Cardiac resynchronization by pacing: an electrical treatment of heart failure. Int J Cardiol 2004;94:151–61.

79. Daniel WG, Erbel R, Kasper W, et al. Safety of transesophageal echocardiography: a multicenter survey of 10,419 examinations. Circulation 1991;83:817.

80. Khanderia BK, Seward JB, Tajik AJ. Transesophageal echocardiography. Mayo Clin Proc 1994;69:856.

81. Cheitlin MD, Armstrong WF, Aurigemma GP, et al. ACC/AHA/ASE 2003 guideline update for the clinical application of echocardiography: summary article: a report of the American College of Cardiology/American Heart Association Task Force on Practice Guidelines (acc/aha/ase committee to update the 1997 Guidelines for the Clinical application of echocardiography). Circulation 2003;108:1146.

82. ACCF/ASE/ACEP/ASNC/SCAI/SCCT/SCMR 2007 appropriateness criteria for transthoracic and transesophageal echocardiography: a report of the American College of Cardiology Foundation Quality Strategic Directions Committee Appropriateness Criteria Working Group, American Society of Echocardiography, American College of Emergency Physicians, American Society of Nuclear Cardiology, Society for Cardiovascular Angiography and Interventions, Society of Cardiovascular Computed Tomography, and the Society for Cardiovascular Magnetic Resonance Endorsed by the American College of Chest Physicians and the Society of Critical Care Medicine. J Am Coll Cardiol 2007;50(2): 187–204. Accessed June 2008.

83. Manning W, Kannam JP. Transesophageal echocardiography: technology, complications, indications and normal views. Available at: www.uptodate.com.

84. Min JK, Spencer KT, Furlong KT, et al. Clinical features of complications from transesophageal echocardiography: a single-center case series of 10,000 consecutive examinations. J Am Soc Echocardiogr 2005;18:925.

85. Moore TJ, Walsh CS, Cohen MR, et al. Reported adverse event cases of methemoglobinemia associated with benzocaine products. Arch Intern Med 2004;164: 1192.

86. Henry LR, Pizzini M, Delarso B, et al. Methemoglobinemia: early intraoperative detection by clinical observation. Laryngoscope 2004;114:2025.

Anesthesia in the Cardiac Catheterization Laboratory and Electrophysiology Laboratory

Douglas C. Shook, MD[a],*, Robert M. Savage, MD[b,c]

KEYWORDS

- Anesthesia • Catheterization • Electrophysiology
- Cardiac • Cardiology • Intervention

Procedures and interventions in the cardiac catheterization laboratory (CCL) and electrophysiology laboratory (EPL) are more complex and involve acutely ill patients. Modern procedures take longer to perform, requiring technical precision and greater focus by cardiologists for a successful result. In this new and changing arena, collaboration and planning between cardiologists and anesthesiologists are required for both patient safety and procedural success.

The focus of this article is the transformation of that information into a safe and effective anesthesia management plan for the CCL and EPL.

THE LABORATORY ENVIRONMENT

Becoming familiar with the laboratory workspace and personnel is imperative. Typically there is a control station and procedure room. The control station is shielded from radiation and usually has a technician recording the progress of the procedure. The technician communicates with the cardiologist frequently and controls many aspects of the case, including patient monitoring, video recording and editing, and digital record keeping.

[a] Department of Anesthesiology, Perioperative and Pain Medicine, Brigham and Women's Hospital, Harvard Medical School, 75 Francis Street, Boston, MA 02115, USA
[b] Department of Cardiothoracic Anesthesia and The Cleveland Clinic Foundation, Mail Code G30, 9500 Euclid Avenue, Cleveland, OH 44195, USA
[c] Department of Cardiovascular Medicine, The Cleveland Clinic Foundation, Mail Code G30, 9500 Euclid Avenue, Cleveland, OH 44195, USA
* Corresponding author.
E-mail address: dshook@partners.org (D.C. Shook).

Anesthesiology Clin 27 (2009) 47–56
doi:10.1016/j.anclin.2008.10.011
1932-2275/08/$ – see front matter © 2009 Elsevier Inc. All rights reserved.

The procedure room is where the cardiologist, anesthesiologist, nurses, and other technicians care for the patient during the procedure. Equipment in the procedure room includes fluoroscopy, the procedure table, screens for viewing the procedure, a sterile table for the cardiologist, storage of various catheters and wires for the procedure, and blood analysis machines. The anesthesiologist should become familiar with what each room contains, and particularly the location of gas outlets and suction, monitors for vital signs, cardioverter/defibrillator, emergency medications, and any airway equipment normally stored in the room. The anesthesiologist may need to familiarize him/herself with different brands of equipment not found in the operating room. Locations for a ventilator, anesthesia cart, and possibly a fiberoptic cart also should be planned if needed. Other equipment regularly used during cases includes ventricular assist devices and echocardiography.

Most CCLs and EPLs are designed for the cardiologist and not for the needs of the anesthesiologist. Space always is an issue in complex cases. Collaboration and preprocedure planning are essential. The fluoroscopy table and fluoroscopy equipment are controlled by the cardiologist and can move unexpectedly during the procedure. Long intravenous lines, extra oxygen tubing, and long breathing circuits must be used to allow movement of both the table and fluoroscopy equipment.

Basic monitoring equipment for sedation or regional or general anesthesia may not be present in the CCL and EPL. Assisting with a sedation issue during a procedure can be more difficult if end-tidal CO_2 is not being monitored. Having end-tidal CO_2 monitors in all rooms is important for safe patient care. Because an anesthesia workroom typically is not located near the CCL or EPL, stocking laboratories with airway equipment and an emergency airway cart is essential. Having an anesthesia cart stocked with extra intravenous (IV) lines, medications, and other items located in the CCL and EPL helps during emergent consultations. All personnel in the laboratory should know the location of this equipment, because the anesthesiologist will not have time to gather the equipment if called emergently to a procedure area.

ANESTHESIA CONSULTATION

There are no established guidelines for anesthesia consultation in the CCL and EPL. Many emergencies are avoided by preprocedure planning of patient sedation or advising that general anesthesia should be considered. Consultation is based either on patient factors or procedure complexity.

Patient airway factors that should trigger an anesthesia consultation include morbid obesity, obstructive sleep apnea, inability to lie flat, and known or suspected difficult airways (Mallampati class III or IV). Personnel in the preprocedure area should be taught how to perform basic airway histories and examinations to establish whether consultation should be obtained. Other patient factors that may trigger an anesthesia consultation include chronic obstructive pulmonary disease, low oxygen saturation, current congestive heart failure, hemodynamic instability, psychiatric disorders, and any medications that could complicate the administration of sedative agents.

Procedure factors that may prompt a provider to seek an anesthesia consultation include the potential for an outcome that requires immediate surgical back-up such as unprotected left-main coronary artery stenting or investigational percutaneous valve procedures. These procedures typically are longer and more complex, requiring the focused attention of the cardiologist. Complex arrhythmia ablation procedures, complicated lead extractions (laser lead extraction), and biventricular pacemaker procedures also should have anesthesia consultations. Any procedure that requires general anesthesia needs preprocedure anesthesia evaluation.

Establishing criteria for anesthesia consultation eventually will lead to more efficient and safer patient care. Better preprocedure planning can take place, such as route of catheterization (radial versus femoral), avoiding oversedation in susceptible patients, planned elevation of the patient's head during the procedure to alleviate sedation-induced airway obstruction, and having continuous positive airway pressure available for patients who have known or suspected obstructive sleep apnea. Personnel delivering sedation will be more comfortable caring for the patient, cardiologists can focus on the task at hand, and anesthesiologists are alerted to the possible complications they may be called to manage.

THE PATIENT

If an anesthesia consultation is warranted, a comprehensive preprocedure evaluation is essential. A complete history includes not only the typical evaluation questions but also a comprehensive review of all previous cardiac interventions (diagnostic catheterizations, stent placement and location, left- and right-sided cardiac pressures, surgical interventions, arrhythmia interventions and ablations), echocardiograms (ventricular function and dimensions, valve disease), chest radiographs, and any recent changes in the patient's medication regimen.

Many patients arrive in the preprocedure area after failed interventions, recent myocardial infarctions, acute exacerbations of heart failure, or with uncontrolled arrhythmias. These patients are not the typical patient population cared for in the operating rooms, because operations for most of these patients would be cancelled using the current American College of Cardiology/American Heart Association guidelines for preoperative assessment.[1] Awareness of the patient's current state of health is imperative. In some cases, the anesthesiologists may be the only care provider to be aware of recent changes is health status, because of the urgency and focus of the intervention at hand.

Determining the urgency of the procedure in relation to anesthetic needs and procedural complications requires communication with the CCL and EPL teams. The condition of some patients can be optimized before the procedure to avoid general anesthesia. For example, improving diuresis and adjusting medication regimens to optimize respiratory function, thereby permitting the patient to lie flat comfortably during the procedure, can increase the probability of a successful result. Radial artery catheterization instead of a femoral approach may be a better option in some patients, because this approach allows the patient to sit in a more upright position during the procedure. Some patients need the procedure emergently, limiting options and requiring the direct involvement of an anesthesiologist for sedation or general anesthesia.

Emergently managing an airway in a sedated patient in the CCL and EPL can be difficult. The fluoroscopy table is different from an operating room table. The head of the bed cannot be elevated, and the cardiologist has the table controls. In addition, the fluoroscopy equipment usually surrounds the patient's head, limiting access; the patient may be hemodynamically unstable, further complicating airway management. Finally, personnel in the CCL and EPL do not have training in advance airway management and can be of little help in an emergency.

Therefore, airway assessment is critical in this environment. Ease of endotracheal intubation should be assessed and also the ability to mask ventilate should be evaluated, because mask ventilation can bridge a moment of oversedation during a procedure. Langeron and colleagues[2] identified five independent criteria associated with difficult mask ventilation: age greater than 55 years, body mass index greater than 26, presence of a beard, lack of teeth, and history of snoring. The presence of two of these factors indicates possible difficult mask ventilation. A history of difficult intubation or possible difficult intubation does not preclude sedation but should be a warning that oversedation can be dangerous, and communication with all personnel involved in the procedure is warranted. Everyone should be alerted to the location of airway supplies and early communication of sedation issues during the procedure.

SEDATION

Most procedures in the CCL and EPL are performed using mild to moderate sedation administered by trained personnel and local anesthetic infiltration at the site of catheter placement by the cardiologist. Non-anesthesia personnel administering mild to moderate sedation should be trained in the pharmacology of commonly used agents and be able to recognize and manage respiratory and hemodynamic indicators for mild, moderate, and deep sedation.[3] Personnel administering sedative agents should be able to manage the next level of sedation safely. The possible synergistic drug interactions of benzodiazepines, opioids, and other commonly administered sedatives such as diphenhydramine (given to patients who have IV contrast reactions) must be well understood, especially in patients who have complicated airways or diminished respiratory capacity. Anesthesiologists should take an active role in developing and maintaining sedation standards for non-anesthesia personnel throughout the hospital.[3]

Patients in the CCL and EPL commonly are sedated with fentanyl and midazolam because of the ease of drug titration and their shorter redistribution and elimination half-lives. In patients who have complicated airways, obstructive symptoms, or respiratory or hemodynamic compromise, minimal sedation usually is recommended with liberal use of local anesthesia for patient comfort. Patient anxiety and fear can be treated with verbal comfort, reassurance, and a small amount of midazolam. Avoiding fentanyl eliminates the synergistic respiratory depressant effect, and most pain is alleviated once local anesthesia has been administered.

The anesthesiologist has a greater medication arsenal available for complicated patients and procedures. Management of sedation requires a complete understanding of the procedure, in addition to the patient's comorbidities. Tachypnea and tachycardia from light sedation can be just as dangerous as airway obstruction and snoring from deep sedation. Both can make an intervention more difficult for the cardiologist. In many instances, deep sedation, a situation that is ideally suited for the assistance of an anesthesiologist, is necessary only for a couple of minutes during a procedure (eg, testing an implantable cardioverter-defibrillator [ICD] after implantation).

Dexmedetomidine (an α_2-agonist) may be ideal in certain patients in the CCL who have complicated airways or mild respiratory compromise, because less respiratory depression is associated with its administration.[4] In patients in the EPL, dexmedetomidine may not be appropriate because it causes sympatholysis, which can be a problem when trying to induce arrhythmias for either diagnosis or treatment (ablation).

Sometimes, because of the complexity of the procedure and/or respiratory and airway compromise of the patient, sedation is not appropriate, and general anesthesia is administered. In most instances, it is safer to start a procedure with general anesthesia than to convert during the procedure.

MONITORING

Just as the room set-up in the CCL and EPL is designed for the cardiologist, so is patient monitoring. The fluoroscopy screen and patient vital signs are easy for the cardiologist to see but may be difficult for the anesthesiologist to see if he/she is at the head of the bed. Establishing the best location to view the necessary monitors is essential and may require changing the current room set-up. Being able to see the fluoroscopy screen is helpful to monitor the progress of the procedure and anticipate changes in hemodynamics or patient comfort.

Certain simple functions such as blood pressure cuff cycling and pulse oximetry volume typically are controlled outside the actual procedure room; if so, the anesthesiologist may want to add his/her own equipment. In addition, for prolonged cases in compromised patients, invasive arterial monitoring that is visible to the anesthesiologist may be important, because the blood pressure cuff may not function during fast or erratic heart rhythms. Invasive arterial monitoring is available in many cases, because arterial access is necessary to perform the procedure, but it may be difficult for the anesthesiologist to see the waveform unless an effort is made to display it on the anesthesia machine or other equipment close to the anesthesiologist. Some CCLs and EPLs may not have end-tidal CO_2 monitoring readily available. End-tidal CO_2 monitoring is not required for sedation cases but is recommended, especially for patients who will need deep sedation.[3] The American Society of Anesthesiologists has established monitoring guidelines for sedation by anesthesia and non-anesthesia personnel in non–operating room locations.[3,5]

In many cases transesophageal echocardiography (TEE) is used to guide and monitor the patient during the procedure. Familiarity with standard views and assessment of cardiac function assists the anesthesiologist in determining the progress of the case, including success and complications of the procedure. If hemodynamic instability occurs, TEE provides instant assessment of contractility, volume status, and valve function. Positioning the TEE screen so that it is visible to the cardiologist performing the procedure as well as to the anesthesiologist performing the TEE can be helpful.

MEDICATIONS

In addition to the standard medications used for sedation and general anesthesia, the anesthesiologist must be familiar with the pharmacokinetics and pharmacodynamics of medications commonly used in both the CCL and EPL. Medications include heparin, glycoprotein IIb/IIIa platelet receptor inhibitors, clopidogrel, direct thrombin inhibitors such as bivalirudin, and vasoactive and inotropic medications. In addition, many patients in the EPL are treated with antiarrhythmic agents of a variety of classes. Common medications include sodium-channel blockers (class 1: quinidine, lidocaine, flecainide), β-blockers (class 2: metoprolol, sotalol), potassium-channel blockers (class 3: amiodarone, sotalol, ibutilide, dofetilide), and calcium-channel blockers (class 4: verapamil, diltiazem).

Before the procedure, it must be made clear who will deliver medications to the patient. The cardiologist usually has the nurse in the room administer drugs such as heparin and vasoactive and inotropic medications. In addition, the cardiologist may administer bolus medications such as nitroglycerine or calcium-channel blockers directly into cardiac catheters; these medications can have a profound effect on the patient's hemodynamics. The anesthesiologist must be informed before the administration of boluses so that subsequent hemodynamic effects can be anticipated.

SPECIFIC ANESTHETIC CONSIDERATIONS

As mentioned earlier, the anesthesiologist must understand the procedure completely to be able to anticipate the patient's anesthetic needs. This section describes some of the anesthetic implications that should be anticipated. The considerations of room set-up, availability of anesthesia equipment, patient evaluation, and medication administration described earlier apply to each of these situations.

Percutaneous Coronary Interventions

Percutaneous coronary interventions commonly are performed using mild to moderate sedation under the direction of the cardiologist. Anesthesia involvement typically occurs in patients presenting with respiratory insufficiency, hemodynamic compromise, or emergently during the procedure because of sedation complications or acute patient decompensation. Close communication with the cardiologist is imperative, because management decisions usually need to be made expeditiously. Information such as recently administered medications, IV access, invasive monitoring, and stage of the procedure must be obtained. Access to the patient's head can be difficult, as mentioned previously. If an airway must be established, priority needs to be given to the anesthesiologist, and the table and fluoroscopy equipment may need to be moved temporarily. Placement of an endotracheal tube is preferred to a laryngeal mask airway. In general, the use of a laryngeal mask airway is not recommended in the CCL and EPL because it can be dislodged by the constant moving of the fluoroscopy equipment and table. In addition, patients can become acutely unstable, and having an endotracheal tube in place eliminates the need to manage an airway further during a crisis.

Percutaneous Ventricular Assist Devices

Percutaneous ventricular assist devices (TandemHeart, Cardiac Assist, Inc., Pittsburg, Pennsylvania, and Impella Recover LP 2.5 and 5.0, Abiomed Inc, Danvers, Massachusetts) are placed in patients undergoing high-risk percutaneous coronary interventions (unprotected left main) or high-risk ablation procedures or who are hemodynamically compromised (cardiogenic shock).[6–8] The anesthesiologist usually is consulted for these procedures because the patient already is unstable or because the procedure can have both airway and hemodynamic complications. Depending on the procedure and state of the patient, either sedation or general anesthesia can be used to care for the patient safely. Communication with the cardiologist helps determine the type of anesthetic most appropriate for the case.

The TandemHeart and Impella LP 5.0 can produce cardiac outputs that can completely replace left ventricular function. During this time, pulse oximetry and non-invasive blood pressure cuffs may not work properly, because blood flow may not be pulsatile. The Impella LP 2.5 uses a smaller cannula that achieves a maximum cardiac output of 2.5 L/min. The patient must have some intrinsic cardiac function to maintain hemodynamic stability.

Invasive monitoring is available because arterial cannulation is used during the procedure. Large-bore IV access is desirable because a large amount of blood loss is possible during the procedure.[9] Blood loss is more likely with the TandemHeart or Impella LP 5.0, because larger cannulas are used. Surgical back-up usually is necessary during these procedures. The anesthesiologist should confirm that back-up is available.

Percutaneous Closure of Septal Defects

Percutaneous closure procedures are used to close patent foramen ovale, atrial septal defects (ASD) and ventricular septal defects (VSD). Patient history is important to determine the reason for closing the defect. Closure of a patent foramen ovale tends to be simpler than closure of an ASD. In patients who have ASDs, it is important to determine if right ventricular function and pulmonary arterial pressures are normal, because the right side of the heart has been volume overloaded by the typical left-to-right shunt through the ASD. In patients who have VSDs, the anesthesiologist needs to determine if the VSD is congenital or acquired (post–myocardial infraction) and the direction of flow through the defect. Typically VSDs have left-to-right flow. Patients who have post–myocardial infarction VSDs can be hemodynamically unstable and may be more likely to have complications (hypotension, arrhythmias) during closure of the defect.[10,11] Complications that can occur during the placement of any device in the CCL include air embolism, device embolization, malposition, thrombosis and embolization (pulmonary or systemic), arrhythmias (arteriovenous nodal block), hypotension, valve dysfunction, and cardiac perforation.[9,11–13]

Echocardiography is used during the procedure to help guide placement and confirm a successful result. If TEE is used, general anesthesia will be necessary for the procedure. Intracardiac echocardiography also can be used to guide the procedure. If intracardiac echocardiography is used, the procedure can be performed under sedation.[14] The choice of sedation or general anesthesia should be based on the complexity of the closure and the patient's medical history.

Arterial access by the cardiologist may not be necessary for the procedure. If invasive arterial monitoring is needed (in VSD closures), a radial arterial line should be placed. Given the possible complications, two IVs should be placed so that one can be used for boluses and the other for infusions. The cardiologist can place a femoral venous line for infusions if necessary.

Percutaneous Valve Repair and Replacement

Although all percutaneous valve repairs and replacements are investigational, they represent the changing paradigm of interventional cardiology procedures: the procedures are more complex and are performed in more acutely ill patients. Medical and surgical approaches to the care of complex cardiac patient now share common ground. The anesthesiologist needs to be prepared for this new and changing patient population.

All percutaneous mitral valve repairs are performed under general anesthesia with fluoroscopic and TEE guidance. Patients typically have moderate to severe mitral regurgitation. The type of device and approach should be communicated before the procedure.[15,16]

During these cases, the procedure room is very crowded, and establishing space to care for the patient can be difficult. Two peripheral IVs should be placed for infusions and boluses. Endotracheal intubation is preferred, and arterial invasive monitoring should be considered, depending on the patient's ventricular function. Communication during the procedure is vital for successful placement of the device, because the procedure can be long, and multiple attempts may be needed to ensure proper device placement with an acceptable result.

Percutaneous aortic valve replacement involves patients who are extremely ill. Patients have severe aortic stenosis, New York Heart Association class IV symptoms, and comorbidities that exclude them from cardiac surgery because of excessive risk.[17] As in percutaneous mitral valve repairs, fluoroscopy and TEE are used to guide device placement. Patients frequently become hemodynamically unstable during the case and can develop myocardial ischemia and significant arrhythmias. Most patients receive general endotracheal anesthesia and invasive monitoring. Central IV access is preferable to infuse necessary medications.

Catheter Ablations

Most catheter ablations are performed with moderate sedation and standard monitoring. Patients can be young and essentially healthy or have extensive comorbidities. Some of the procedures can be very long (6–8 hours) and may require anesthesia consultation to keep the patient comfortable and movement minimized. Coughing, snoring, and partial airway obstruction can be problematic during intracardiac mapping, because they precipitate a swinging motion of the intra-atrial septum and make transseptal catheter placement difficult. Deep sedation sometimes is necessary to keep the patient comfortable during ablations. Drugs that affect the sympathetic nervous system should be avoided, if possible, during mapping of ectopic foci and tracts. In patients who have ventricular dysfunction, inotropic and vasoactive agents may be necessary both to sedate the patient and to maintain hemodynamic stability during arrhythmia induction.[9] Communication with the cardiologist is necessary in these situations to maintain patient safety and still allow the mapping process to proceed. Frequently, electrical cardioversion is necessary during the case, and deep sedation may be required for the patient to tolerate the delivered shock. Usually 20 to 40 mg of propofol is all that is needed to accomplish temporary deeper sedation.

Implantable Cardioverter-Defibrillators and Biventricular Pacemakers

Many patients receiving ICDs or biventricular pacemakers have multiple comorbidities including a history of ventricular tachycardia/fibrillation, an ejection fraction less than 30%, and coronary artery disease, because these conditions are indications for ICD placement.[18,19] Other indications include arrhythmogenic right ventricular dysplasia, long QT syndrome, and hypertrophic cardiomyopathy.[19]

Most of these devices are placed with mild to moderate sedation and standard monitors. Testing the device requires deep sedation or general anesthesia. ICD placement and testing can be accomplished without an arterial line. External cardioverter/defibrillator pads are placed on the patient at the beginning of the procedure. When testing ICDs, the pads are used induce ventricular fibrillation and to serve as back-up if the implanted device fails.

Typically an implanted ICD is tested twice at the end of the procedure. Repeated testing usually is well tolerated without deterioration of ventricular function even in patients who have ejection fractions of less than 35%.[20,21] In patients who have evidence of untreated coronary disease, recent stent placement, or evidence of atrial or ventricular thrombus, testing sometimes is omitted. Significant coronary artery disease is a concern when testing, because prolonged hypotension is a possible complication. It is important to remember that ICD testing always is an elective procedure should the patient demonstrate deterioration during implantation.[9]

In some patients who need ICDs, biventricular pacemakers also are placed for cardiac resynchronization therapy. Any patient scheduled for placement of a biventricular pacemaker has extensive cardiac morbidity. These patients have low ejection fractions and associated comorbidities including valvular heart disease, pulmonary hypertension, and right ventricular dysfunction. Patients may not be able to lie flat comfortably and easily become hemodynamically unstable with sedation. Oversedation can lead to hypercapnia that may not be tolerated in patients who have pulmonary hypertension and/or right ventricular dysfunction. The anesthesiologist must be ready to convert to general anesthesia at any time during the case. The placement of a coronary sinus lead for biventricular pacing can be difficult, making the procedure much longer than dual-chamber pacemaker and ICD placements. Complications from these procedures include possible cardiac injury (perforation/tamponade), myocardial infarction, stroke, and pneumothorax from the subclavian venous access.

RADIATION

Anesthesiologists typically come to the CCL or EPL and must dig through the available lead aprons worn by other members of the CCL or EPL team who are not present that day. They may take shortcuts regarding radiation protection because anesthesiologists have not spent much time in fluoroscopy rooms on a regular basis. Many of the cases described have significant radiation exposure during the procedure.

All radiation exposure should be as low as reasonably achievable during the procedure.[22] Reductions in radiation time, distance from the source of radiation, and barriers to radiation are the three mechanisms for reducing exposure. Radiation time is under the control of the cardiologist performing the procedure. Many of the new and more complex procedures (device placement, percutaneous valves, biventricular pacemakers, ablations) can result in prolonged exposure to radiation.

The distance from the source of radiation and barriers to radiation are under the control of the anesthesiologist. The radiation beam attenuates according to the inverse square law $(1/d^2)$.[22] The strength of the beam decreases exponentially with the distance from the radiation source. Barriers such as lead aprons and thyroid collars should be worn at all times. Even with proper leaded apparel, 18% of active bone marrow is exposed to the effects of radiation.[23] Lead shields should be used for additional protection. The use of leaded eyeglasses is highly recommended to reduce the risk of cataracts. Every anesthesiologist spending time in the CCL or EPL should wear a dosimeter to track cumulative radiation exposure. A study by Katz[23] in 2005 demonstrated that radiation exposure to an anesthesia department doubled after the introduction of an EPL.[23]

SUMMARY

The anesthesiologists' patient safety record in the operating rooms is well documented. Safely caring for this growing patient population in the CCL and EPL is now a concern for all anesthesiologists and cardiologists. Anesthesiologists are uniquely trained to care for this complex patient population, allowing the cardiologist to focus on completing the interventional procedure successfully. Anesthesiologists, in collaboration with the cardiologists, must establish guidelines for their involvement in patient care and procedure planning in the CCL and EPL.

REFERENCES

1. Fleisher LA, Beckman JA, Brown KA, et al. ACC/AHA 2007 guidelines on perioperative cardiovascular evaluation and care for noncardiac surgery: executive summary: a report of the American college of cardiology/American heart association task force on practice guidelines (writing committee to revise the 2002 guidelines on perioperative cardiovascular evaluation for noncardiac surgery). Anesth Analg 2008;106:685–712.
2. Langeron O, Masso E, Huraux C, et al. Prediction of difficult mask ventilation. Anesthesiology 2000;92:1229–36.
3. American Society of Anesthesiologists Task Force on Sedation and Analgesia by Non-Anesthesiologists. Practice guidelines for sedation and analgesia by non-anesthesiologists. Anesthesiology 2002;96:1004–17.
4. Paris A, Tonner PH. Dexmedetomidine in anaesthesia. Curr Opin Anaesthesiol 2005;18:412–8.
5. ASA guidelines for nonoperating room anesthetizing locations. Available at: http://www.asahq.org/publicationsAndServices/standards/14.pdf. Accessed August 27, 2008.
6. Henriques JP, Remmelink M, Baan J Jr, et al. Safety and feasibility of elective high-risk percutaneous coronary intervention procedures with left ventricular support of the Impella Recover LP 2.5. Am J Cardiol 2006;97:990–2.

7. Kar B, Adkins LE, Civitello AB, et al. Clinical experience with the TandemHeart percutaneous ventricular assist device. Tex Heart Inst J 2006;33:111–5.
8. Pretorius M, Hughes AK, Stahlman MB, et al. Placement of the TandemHeart percutaneous left ventricular assist device. Anesth Analg 2006;103:1412–3.
9. Shook DC, Gross W. Offsite anesthesiology in the cardiac catheterization lab. Curr Opin Anaesthesiol 2007;20:352–8.
10. Martinez MW, Mookadam F, Sun Y, et al. Transcatheter closure of ischemic and post-traumatic ventricular septal ruptures. Catheter Cardiovasc Interv 2007;69: 403–7.
11. Garay F, Cao QL, Hjazi ZM. Percutaneous closure of post-myocardial infarction ventricular septal defect. J Interv Cardiol 2006;19:S67–72.
12. Carroll JD, Dodge S, Groves BM. Percutaneous patent foramen ovale closure. Cardiol Clin 2005;23:13–33.
13. Nugent AW, Britt A, Gauvreau K, et al. Device closure rates of simple atrial septal defects optimized by the STARFlex device. J Am Coll Cardiol 2006;48:538–44.
14. Boccalandro F, Baptista E, Muench A, et al. Comparison of intracardiac echocardiography versus transesophageal echocardiography guidance for percutaneous transcatheter closure of atrial septal defect. Am J Cardiol 2004;93:437–40.
15. Block PC. Percutaneous transcatheter repair for mitral regurgitation. J Interv Cardiol 2006;19:547–51.
16. Feldman T. Percutaneous mitral valve repair. J Interv Cardiol 2007;20:488–94.
17. Rajagopal V, Kapadia SR, Tuzcu EM. Advances in the percutaneous treatment of aortic and mitral valve disease. Minerva Cardioangiol 2007;55:83–94.
18. Moss AJ, Zareba W, Hall WJ, et al. Prophylactic implantation of a defibrillator in patients with myocardial infarction and reduced ejection fraction. N Engl J Med 2002;346:877–83.
19. Epstein AE, DiMarco JP, Ellenbogen KA, et al. ACC/AHA/HRS 2008 guidelines for device-based therapy of cardiac rhythm abnormalities: a report of the American college of cardiology/American heart association task force on practice guidelines (writing committee to revise the ACC/AHA/NASPE 2002 guideline update for implantation of cardiac pacemakers and antiarrhythmia devices) developed in collaboration with the American Association for Thoracic Surgery and Society of Thoracic Surgeons. J Am Coll Cardiol 2008;51:e1–62.
20. Meyer J, Mollhoff T, Seifert T, et al. Cardiac output is not affected during intraoperative testing of the automatic implantable cardioverter defibrillator. J Cardiovasc Electrophysiol 1996;7:211–6.
21. Gilbert TB, Gold MR, Shorofsky SR, et al. Cardiovascular responses to repetitive defibrillation during implantable cardioverter-defibrillator testing. J Cardiothorac Vasc Anesth 2002;16:180–5.
22. Bashore TM, Bates ER, Berger PB, et al. American college of cardiology/society for cardiac angiography and interventions clinical expert consensus document on cardiac catheterization laboratory standards. A report of the American college of cardiology task force on clinical expert consensus documents. J Am Coll Cardiol 2001;37:2170–214.
23. Katz JD. Radiation exposure to anesthesia personnel: the impact of an electrophysiology laboratory. Anesth Analg 2005;101:1725–6.

Anesthesiology and Gastroenterology

Willem J.S. de Villiers, MD, PhD, MHCM

KEYWORDS

- Gastroenterologist-directed propofol • NOTES • Halo system
- Endoscopic mucosal resection • Deep balloon enteroscopy
- Chromoendoscopy

Sedation and analgesia are considered by many gastroenterologists to be integral components of the endoscopic examination. For example, more than 98% of endoscopists in the United States routinely administer sedation during upper and lower endoscopies.[1] Sedation is intended primarily to reduce a patient's anxiety and discomfort, consequently improving their tolerability and satisfaction for the procedure. Endoscopic sedation also minimizes a patient's risk of physical injury during an examination and provides the endoscopist with an ideal environment for a thorough examination. Despite the benefits of sedation, its use remains problematic. Sedation delays patient recovery and discharge, adds to the overall cost of an endoscopic procedure, and increases the risk of cardiopulmonary complications. Notwithstanding these considerations, the use of sedation during endoscopy continues to increase throughout the world.[1,2]

The high costs of providing anesthesia by specialists and the relative lack of specialist personnel in many countries have led to the wider introduction of sedation delivered by nonanesthesiologists. Such sedation should be targeted for moderate levels of sedation; however, personnel should be able to avoid—and rescue patients from—deeper sedation levels. Several conditions have to be fulfilled to provide proper and safe nonanesthesiologist sedation for endoscopy, especially when propofol is to be used. These conditions include formal training, supervision by anesthesiology staff, and the definition of standard operating procedures on the national as well as local levels.

The goal of this review is (1) to provide a gastroenterology perspective on the use of propofol in gastroenterology endoscopic practice, and (2) to describe newer GI endoscopy procedures that gastroenterologists perform that might involve anesthesiologists. Mutual understanding and respect are fundamental requirements for the

Division of Digestive Diseases and Nutrition, Department of Internal Medicine, University of Kentucky Medical Center, University of Kentucky College of Medicine, 800 Rose Street, Room MN649, Lexington, KY 40536, USA
E-mail address: willem.devilliers@uky.edu

Anesthesiology Clin 27 (2009) 57–70
doi:10.1016/j.anclin.2008.10.007
1932-2275/08/$ – see front matter © 2009 Elsevier Inc. All rights reserved.

integration of gastrointestinal endoscopy and anesthesia services to optimize patient outcomes.

PROPOFOL USE IN GI ENDOSCOPY

The acceptance of colonoscopy as the gold standard modality to screen for colorectal polyps and cancer has dramatically increased the number of these procedures performed annually. There has also been an increasing emphasis on factors that could improve patient acceptance of the procedure and patient satisfaction as well as efficiency and throughput in endoscopy centers. Propofol initially was developed and approved in 1989 as a hypnotic agent for induction and maintenance of anesthesia. Accordingly, its US Food and Drug Administration (FDA) product label states "[propofol] should be administered only by persons trained in the administration of general anesthesia."[3] Since approval in the late 1980s, its clinical applications have expanded to include monitored anesthesia care and procedural sedation. Compared with conventional endoscopic sedation, it is generally accepted that propofol offers faster and more complete patient recovery, greater endoscopist and patient satisfaction, and better success with the hard-to-sedate patient.

Worldwide, the experience with gastroenterologist-directed administration of propofol now exceeds 200,000 patient experiences with no mortalities.[4–7] This, combined with improvements in our understanding of its dosing and titration for moderate sedation, have prompted several professional medical societies to question the medical necessity of restricting its use to anesthesiology professionals. The American Gastroenterological Association, the American College of Gastroenterology, and the American Society for Gastrointestinal Endoscopy all support gastroenterologist-directed administration of propofol by gastroenterologists. In a joint statement, the three societies declared that "with adequate training, physician-supervised nurse administration of propofol can be done safely and effectively."[3] However, the American Society for Anesthesiology countered that the use of propofol should be restricted to those experienced in the skills (such as endotracheal intubation) that are required during general anesthesia.[8] Much of this debate, during a time of increasing health care costs and decreasing physician reimbursements, seems to reflect economic rather than clinical concerns.[9]

Two models have emerged for the administration of propofol by endoscopists: nurse-administered propofol sedation (NAPS) and combination propofol sedation (also referred to as gastroenterologist-directed sedation). Both techniques emphasize several key principles: (1) the use of an established protocol for drug administration, (2) a sedation team with appropriate education and training, and (3) continuous patient assessment of clinical and physiologic parameters throughout the procedure.

The practice of NAPS involves a trained registered nurse whose sole responsibilities are patient monitoring and the administration of propofol. Recommendations for the initial bolus of propofol range from 10 to 60 mg, and additional boluses of 10 to 20 mg are administered with a minimum of 20 to 30 seconds between doses. Propofol dosing and the depth of sedation are individualized to the needs of each patient. Because propofol possesses no analgesic effect, many patients receiving NAPS will require deep sedation. Heart rate, blood pressure, and pulse oximetry are monitored routinely during NAPS. In most protocols, supplemental oxygen is administered to all patients.

Rex and colleageus[7] published a retrospective review of more than 36,000 endoscopies performed with NAPS at three centers, two within the United States and one in Switzerland. The targeted depth of sedation was not specified, and the mean doses of propofol at each center were 107, 158, and 245 mg, and 144, 209, and 287 mg, during esophagogastroduodenoscopy and colonoscopy, respectively. The rate of clinically important events, defined as an episode of apnea or other airway compromise requiring assisted ventilation (bag-mask), ranged from approximately 1 per 500 to 1 per 1000. In this large case series, endotracheal intubation was not required and no patient suffered permanent injury or death.

Tohda and colleagues[10] recently reported the results of 27,500 endoscopies performed with NAPS during a 6-year period. These investigators targeted moderate rather than deep sedation. Supplemental oxygen was not provided routinely. The mean doses of propofol during esophagogastroduodenoscopy and colonoscopy were 72 and 94 mg, respectively. Notably, there were no serious cardiopulmonary events in this series, and no patient required mask ventilation, endotracheal intubation, or any form of resuscitation.

GASTROENTEROLOGIST-DIRECTED PROPOFOL SEDATION

In combination propofol sedation, also known as gastroenterologist-directed propofol sedation, the dosing responsibility is shared between the physician and nurse, and propofol is combined with very small doses of a benzodiazepine and opioid narcotic.[11] It is thus possible to maximize the desirable therapeutic actions of each agent while minimizing the likelihood of a dose-related adverse reaction. When propofol is combined with small doses of an opioid analgesic and a benzodiazepine, analgesia and amnesia can be achieved with subhypnotic doses of propofol, eliminating the need for deep sedation. Furthermore, more precise dose titration is possible with smaller bolus doses of propofol (5–15 mg), and the potential for pharmacologic reversibility is retained using naloxone or flumazenil. Therefore, combination propofol provides the benefits of propofol-mediated sedation while reducing the risk of rapid, irreversible oversedation.[12]

The published protocols for combination propofol sedation all include a preinduction dose of either an opioid (fentanyl, 25–75 µg; meperidine, 25–50 mg), a benzodiazepine (midazolam, 0.5–2.5 mg), or both.[5,11] An induction dose of propofol then is administered (5–15 mg), followed by additional boluses of 5 to 15 mg titrated to effect. Most protocols target moderate rather than deep sedation. A nurse has primary responsibility for monitoring the patient; however, in contrast with NAPS, both the nurse and the endoscopist participate in all dosing decisions that involve propofol. Furthermore, the nurse responsible for sedation also may perform brief, interruptible tasks such as assisting with tissue acquisition. Clinical and physiologic parameters are monitored in all cases, and in some instances capnography is used as well. Several studies have reported results using a multidrug regimen. These and other studies support the observation that propofol, combined with an opioid and benzodiazepine, is an effective and safe method of sedation when administered by an endoscopist with adequate training.[11]

There is widespread belief among gastroenterologists that propofol provides better sedation for endoscopy than an opioid/benzodiazepine combination. Its benefits over traditional sedation agents are believed to include faster recovery, improved sedation effect, and greater efficiency within the endoscopy unit. Although comparative trials have shown propofol's clear-cut superiority in terms of recovery time and physician satisfaction, similar improvement in patient satisfaction has been more difficult to prove.

MEDICAL AND LEGAL IMPLICATIONS OF PROPOFOL

Although propofol has been used safely and effectively under the direction of endoscopists to provide sedation during endoscopy, the FDA-restricted product label has deterred many gastroenterologists because of concerns about potential liability for medical malpractice.[1] In most jurisdictions, FDA-approved product labels are admissible as evidence in court, so a jury would be allowed to weigh the off-label nature of gastroenterologist-directed propofol sedation. A product label alone generally is insufficient to establish the standard of care (the FDA does not regulate the practice of medicine), but it would be considered by a jury alongside expert testimony. Moreover, many jurisdictions observe the respectable minority rule, which holds that there may be multiple appropriate approaches to a particular medical problem. Numerous clinical studies, professional society guidelines, and expert editorial opinions position this as a respectable minority practice.[13] Thus, if undertaken appropriately, gastroenterologist-directed propofol sedation is reasonable from a medical and legal perspective.

Maximizing patient safety and minimizing liability when administering propofol can be accomplished by adhering to five basic principles. First, the gastroenterologist should ensure compliance with prevailing guidelines produced by professional societies as well as laws and regulations imposed by medical boards and/or credentialing bodies. Second, gastroenterologist-directed propofol sedation should be limited to appropriate, relatively low-risk patients. Third, gastroenterologists and staff should be trained in recognition and management of respiratory depression, the pharmacologic properties of propofol, and advanced cardiac life support. Fourth, endoscopy units should be equipped with resuscitation equipment and drugs, and appropriate monitoring equipment. Fifth, the informed consent discussion should inform the patient of risks, benefits, and alternatives (including the option of having propofol administered by an anesthesiologist) to gastroenterologist-directed propofol sedation, and of the qualifications and experience of the endoscopist to administer the medication. In addition, the gastroenterologist should appreciate that increased use of open-access endoscopy, in which the endoscopist may not have meaningful preprocedure contact with the patient, and increased procedure volumes may have a deleterious impact on the delivery of a thorough informed consent process.

FUTURE DIRECTIONS IN ENDOSCOPIC SEDATION

Several other innovative modalities for drug delivery to patients are being developed for endoscopic sedation. In patient-controlled analgesia/sedation (PCA/S), patient-controlled drug delivery enables the patient to control the timing of medication administration. Colonoscopy, characterized by brief periods of intense discomfort related to stretching or distension of the colon wall, would appear to be ideally suited to this method. Propofol, either alone or combined with an opioid narcotic, is the drug used most often, and multiple trials have shown that PCA/S is safe and effective for endoscopic sedation.[14,15]

On the basis of published studies, several conclusions about PCA/S and endoscopy can be drawn. First, patients receiving PCA/S experience procedure-related satisfaction that is at least comparable with, and in some cases better than, conventional sedation. Second, recovery is faster with PCA/S because the total drug dose usually is reduced. Third, PCA/S may not be suitable for all persons because it requires both the willingness and capacity to comply with instructions. Several patient characteristics have been shown to predict poor tolerance for PCA/S, including young age, female sex, and increased preprocedural anxiety.

A target-controlled infusion (TCI) system is designed to deliver an intravenous drug using an infusion pump and a computer.[16] The computer, programmed with a drug-specific, population-based pharmacokinetic model, calculates the infusion rate that is necessary to achieve the target or desired drug concentration in the blood. The computer signals the infusion pump to deliver the amount of drug necessary to achieve the predetermined drug concentration. This method of TCI, designed to deliver a target concentration of a drug that has been selected by a physician, is referred to as *open-loop* because there is no feedback from the patient. A related *closed-loop* system uses feedback from a real-time measure of drug effect such as muscle relaxation, auditory evoked potential, or another measure of sedation to regulate the concentration of delivered drug. This system should provide sedation that is more individualized, reducing the potential for undersedation and oversedation. The use of TCI, both open- and closed-loop systems, has been studied during endoscopy. The quality of sedation was considered excellent by both endoscopists and nurses. Patient satisfaction and recovery times were comparable in the two groups.[17]

Computer-assisted personalized sedation is a procedure that uses an investigational device that combines TCI of propofol and a physiologic monitoring unit.[18] The device is programmed to reduce or stop an infusion in response to either a clinical (unresponsiveness to audible/tactile stimuli) or physiologic (oxygen desaturation, hypoventilation) indication of oversedation. When patient responsiveness has returned and the physiologic parameters have been restored to normal, drug delivery is resumed at a reduced maintenance rate, based on a recalculated dosing algorithm. Computer-assisted personalized sedation is designed to deliver propofol safely and effectively when used by a trained physician/nurse team.

The feasibility of computer-assisted personalized sedation was evaluated recently by US and Belgian investigators in two studies using an identical protocol. Preliminary data suggest that computer-assisted personalized sedation may provide endoscopists with the ability to deliver propofol safely and effectively without the assistance of an anesthesia professional. A large, multicenter, pivotal trial is currently in progress.

THE ROLE OF ANESTHESIOLOGY IN CURRENT AND FUTURE GI ENDOSCOPY

The important contribution of anesthesiology in achieving satisfactory patient outcomes in current GI endoscopy is well established. The use of an anesthesia professional should be strongly considered for American Society of Anesthesiologists physical status IV and V patients or for patients undergoing emergency GI endoscopy for hemodynamically significant upper gastrointestinal bleeds. Other possible indications include children, patients with a history of alcohol or substance abuse, pregnancy, morbid obesity, neurologic or neuromuscular disorders, and patients who are uncooperative or delirious. Specific endoscopic procedures that may require an anesthesia specialist include endoscopic retrograde cholangiopancreatography (ERCP), endoscopic ultrasound, and complex, lengthy, and potentially uncomfortable therapeutic procedures such as stent placement in the upper gastrointestinal tract and esophagogastroduodenoscopy with drainage of a pseudocyst. These indications are described in detail by Goulson and Fragneto in this issue.

An additional important role for anesthesiology is in sedation quality assurance and improvement in practice safety. A system for assessing outcome measures and complications related to sedation should be established at each facility. Currently no set of clinically important quality indicators to assess adequate sedation has been accepted universally. The emphasis is instead on the documentation of sedation-related adverse events: hypoxemia requiring airway intervention, hypotension or bradycardia requiring pharmacologic intervention, pulmonary aspiration, laryngospasm, unanticipated use of reversal agents, and unanticipated hospitalization. All such adverse events as well as near misses should be reported and analyzed to identify and remedy areas of vulnerability.[19]

Digestive endoscopy has rapidly moved from being a primary diagnostic modality to being extensively used as a therapeutic modality in the management of gastrointestinal diseases. Future directions in GI endoscopy illustrate the ongoing evolution of the field as a multidisciplinary specialty combining advances in a number of areas (radiology, bioengineering, surgery, and gastroenterology). The complex nature of the following described endoscopic procedures will require the increased involvement of anesthesiology professionals to ensure successful outcomes.

NATURAL ORIFICE TRANSLUMENAL ENDOSCOPIC SURGERY

The area of most intense endoscopic investigation is natural orifice translumenal endoscopic surgery (NOTES), an amalgamation of general surgery and gastroenterology that ushers in an era of incisionless approaches to the peritoneal cavity. This term was invented during the first meeting of the Natural Orifice Surgery Consortium for Assessment and Research in July 2005.[20,21]

Currently, NOTES is performed with commercially available flexible video endoscopes, which are advanced through a natural orifice and used to create a controlled transvisceral incision that offers access to the peritoneal cavity. Once the endoscope is passed into the peritoneal cavity, endoscopic devices are advanced through the endoscope's working channels, allowing visualization and manipulation of abdominal tissues. At the completion of the procedure, the point of peritoneal access is closed using endoscopic devices, and the scope is withdrawn from the natural orifice, obviating the need for abdominal wall incisions.

The first translumenal procedures were performed in a porcine model in 2000, and multiple translumenal interventions have subsequently been completed in animal experiments and reported in abstracts and full-length articles.[21] The most common interventions include gastrojejunostomy, cholecystectomy, ligation and resection of pelvic organs, and abdominal wall hernia repair.[22] Human transgastric intraperitoneal interventions and appendectomies were initiated in India in 2003.[23] Thus far, only a limited number of human NOTES procedures have been reported in the United States, but additional translumenal human procedures have been done around the world.[23–25]

The first published human NOTES procedure described transgastric rescue of a prematurely dislodged percutaneous endoscopic gastrostomy tube.[26] The intervention started with peroral endoscopic dilation of the previous gastrostomy site by using an esophageal dilating balloon. The endoscope was then advanced through the gastrostomy into the peritoneal cavity, free fluid was aspirated from the peritoneal cavity, and a guide wire was passed through the external percutaneous endoscopic gastrostomy site into the peritoneal cavity and grasped with an endoscopic snare. The endoscope, snare, and guide wire were withdrawn into the stomach and out the mouth. The new percutaneous endoscopic gastrostomy tube was inserted over the guide wire by using the standard pull technique.

Two transvaginal, purely endoscopic appendectomies were recently reported by two independent groups of investigators from Germany and India.[23,24] Each group performed an appendectomy by using a standard flexible gastroscope and endoscopic accessories (hot biopsy forceps, needle-knives, endoclips, endoscopic detachable loops). There were no complications, and both patients recovered quickly, with an uneventful follow-up.

Other reported human NOTES interventions were done as hybrid procedures with translumenal incision and advancement of the flexible endoscope into the peritoneal cavity, along with direct laparoscopic visualization. These include two transvaginal and one transgastric appendectomies, seven transvaginal and three transgastric cholecystectomies, 10 transgastric diagnostic peritoneoscopies, and three liver biopsies.[21]

The transgastric peritoneoscopy and liver biopsies were technically simple and safe, and provided information comparable with laparoscopic abdominal exploration.[25] In addition to laparoscopic observation, the transvaginal and transgastric cholecystectomies in human beings also used laparoscopic instruments for gallbladder traction or to facilitate access to the cystic artery and cystic duct. To date no complications have been reported during or after human NOTES procedures.[23–26]

Despite the excitement that NOTES generates simply because of the novel approach it entails, sound arguments exist for its continued development. The potential advantages of NOTES approaches to peritoneal surgical issues include the elimination of skin flora–based surgical-site infections and postoperative incisional hernias, the reduction in incisional pain, and the potential for fewer intra-abdominal adhesions due to smaller access sites. The challenges that must be overcome for NOTES to become universally acceptable include reliable peritoneal access, infection prevention, suturing and anastomosis device development, user-friendly spatial orientation, multitasking platform development, intraperitoneal complication management, and reliable visceral closure. An important consideration also is the level of anesthesia that is required for specific procedures. All these principles are in the midst of intense multicenter research and development. Because NOTES occupies a medical niche that incorporates input from experts in both surgery and gastroenterology, the best training may reside in integrated training from both disciplines. This may indeed signify the end for classical training in each respective field, giving way to one hybridized field of endoscopic surgery.

SPYGLASS DIRECT PANCREATICOBILIARY VISUALIZATION SYSTEM

The SpyGlass direct visualization system (Boston Scientific, Natick, Massachusetts) is a mother–daughter scope system using a standard duodenoscope, a 10-Fr daughter scope/catheter with a 1.2-mm working channel, and a 0.77-mm-diameter fiber optic probe intended to provide direct visualization for diagnostic and therapeutic applications during endoscopic procedures in the pancreaticobiliary system, including the hepatic ducts, to identify stones and strictures.[27,28] Conventional ERCP is conducted by using two-dimensional black-and-white images rendered by fluoroscopy, which can potentially lead to an inaccurate or inconclusive clinical diagnosis, potentially creating the need for additional testing. In early trials using an animal model, the SpyGlass system was effective for access, direct visualization, and biopsy in all bile duct quadrants. In addition, SpyGlass procedures can be performed by a single operator, unlike conventional therapeutic upper endoscopy, which requires an operator and an assistant.

The cholangioscopy procedure with the SpyGlass system is performed with the access-and-delivery catheter positioned just below the operating channel of the duodenoscope. The duodenoscope is positioned in front of the papilla, and a sphincterotomy is performed as necessary. The SpyGlass system is introduced into the therapeutic duodenoscope. The bile duct is cannulated, and the SpyScope catheter is used to guide the SpyGlass visualization probe into the biliary tree. The SpyScope catheter and SpyGlass probe are maneuvered up to the desired area of interest within the duct for direct visualization. In addition, selected ducts and branches of interest can be examined during repeated advancement and withdrawal of the system. A SpyBite biopsy forceps guided by using the SpyScope catheter can be introduced, and an endoscopically guided biopsy can be performed. Also, electrohydraulic lithotripsy can be used as needed via a 3-Fr electrohydraulic lithotripsy probe passed through the 1.2-mm working channel. Once this is completed, a standard stone retrieval basket or balloon is used to clear the duct of any remaining stone fragments.[27,28]

A recent case series compared results of conventional ERCP and single-operator duodenoscope-assisted cholangiopancreatoscopy using the SpyGlass direct visualization system. Direct visualization with SpyGlass altered the clinicians' diagnosis or treatment strategy for 19 of 22 patients who had previously been examined unsuccessfully using ERCP but suspected of harboring malignancy, bile duct strictures, retained bile duct stones, or cystic biliary lesions. Overall, SpyGlass examination with or without biopsy was accomplished without technical difficulty for 20 of the 22 cases.[27,28]

This novel technology now allows direct optical diagnostic and therapeutic means where previously only indirect radiographic imaging was available for intervention guidance. The potential applicability of this technology is expanding as other regions in the human body currently too remote or fragile for standard instrument navigation are being investigated.[29]

BARRX MEDICAL HALO SYSTEM

The HALO system (both HALO 360 and HALO 90; BARRX Medical, Inc., Sunnyvale, California), is a novel device designed to treat and circumferentially ablate the esophageal mucosa of patients who have Barrett's esophagus without harming the underlying tissue layers. Cleared by the US FDA in 2001, the HALO system has been commercially available since January 2005.

Using standard endoscopic techniques with the patient under conscious sedation, the HALO system facilitates rapid ablation of long and short segments of Barrett's esophagus in three steps. Initially, the anatomic landmarks and length of Barrett's epithelium are identified by esophagoscopy. A sizing balloon then is used to measure the inner diameter of the esophagus and select the appropriately sized ablation catheter. Finally, a radiofrequency ablation catheter is deployed, which circumferentially ablates a 3-cm-long segment of Barrett's epithelium in less than 1 second. A consistent ablation depth of less than 1 mm avoids damage to the submucosal tissue layers.[30]

Two recent studies established that use of the HALO system was safe and effective for the treatment of patients with Barrett's esophagus and low- or high-grade dysplasia.[30,31] After two treatment sessions, 10 of 11 patients had a complete response for dysplasia. The patient with persistent dysplasia went from high- to low-grade dysplasia and had only small residual islands of Barrett's mucosa left. In the same patient group, the internal esophageal diameter was identical before treatment and 10 weeks afterward, confirming that radiofrequency ablation, in contrast to other ablative and resective techniques, does not result in significant scarring or structuring. In the largest clinical trial of the HALO system to date, the average procedure time was less than 30 minutes. At the 1-year follow-up assessment, 70% of the patients were free of Barrett's esophagus, and no strictures or buried glands were detected in 3,007 surveillance biopsies.[30–32]

ENDOSCOPIC MUCOSAL RESECTION/ENDOSCOPIC SUBMUCOSAL DISSECTION

Endoscopic mucosal resection has been incorporated in Asia as a curative treatment for superficial carcinomas in the foregut. The technique incorporates accessing mucosal lesions via an endoscope, splitting the mucosal/submucosal plane of a segment of the gastrointestinal tract, and removing the mucosal lesion while preserving the submucosa and adventitia of the hollow viscus. Experience with this technique in Western Europe and the Americas is limited because of infrequent screening and diagnosis of early gastric cancers, compared with Japanese and Korean populations.

The use of endoscopic mucosal resection, however, is increasing outside Asia. Deprez and colleagues[33] describe recent results for more than 170 Belgian patients managed satisfactorily with endoscopic resection of esophageal high-grade dysplasia or squamous cell carcinoma and gastric or Barrett's epithelium high-grade dysplasia or adenocarcinoma. Similar results were seen by Ross and colleagues,[34] who treated 16 patients between 2003 and 2005. Of the patients staged as being T1aN0Mx using pretreatment endoscopic ultrasound and found to have corresponding histopathology, none experienced recurrence at a median follow-up assessment 17 months after treatment, according to surveillance endoscopic biopsies. Ell and colleagues[35] recently reported complete local remission for 99 of 100 patients who underwent endoscopic mucosal resection for mucosally based early esophageal adenocarcinoma. Although 11% experienced recurrent or metachronous lesions in the 3 years after treatment, all of these patients were treated successfully with repeat endoscopic resection.

Innovative devices have furthered this relatively young technology, and Seewald and colleagues[36] describe their initial experience with the newly introduced Duette Multiband Mucosectomy Kit (Cook Ireland Ltd., Limerick, Ireland) for the treatment of extensive early esophageal squamous cell carcinoma. The device allows for repeated ligation and resection of targeted mucosal regions without removal and reinsertion of the endoscope. Five patients with more than hemicircumferential involvement of the esophageal wall and a mean involved length of 2.8 cm were successfully treated in one session using endoscopic mucosal resection. Posttreatment stricture was successfully treated using bougienage, and no recurrences were noted 1 year after treatment.

In addition, a modified rigid endoscopic device for suction resection of mucosal lesions (Karl Storz GmbH, Tuttlingen, Germany) is being introduced. This device operates by suctioning a large mucosal area against a transparent and perforated hemicylindrical window. Mucosal resection is performed by using an electrical wire loop at a constant depth of 1 mm. Jaquet and colleagues[37] performed endoscopic mucosal resection in a series of animal trials using hemicircumferential and circumferential mucosectomies 2 to 6 cm long. The deep resection margin of the specimens was noted to be located precisely at the submucosal level.

Despite the seemingly straightforward objectives of endoscopic mucosal resection, difficulty in correctly assessing the depth of tumor invasion and an increase in local recurrence have been reported in cases of large lesions because such lesions often are resected piecemeal. An innovation on standard endoscopic mucosal resection termed *endoscopic submucosal dissection* allows direct dissection of the submucosa and en bloc resection of large lesions. Endoscopic submucosal dissection is not limited by resection size, however. It still is associated with a higher incidence of complications than endoscopic mucosal resection and requires a high level of endoscopic skill.[38]

Endoscopic submucosal dissection allows for the same approach as that used for mucosal resection, except that the deeper submucosal tissue plane is opened with the aid of tissue elevation using solutions such as saline, glycerol, sodium hyaluronate, or fructose immediately before the dissection. Although technically demanding, endoscopic submucosal dissection is quite effective. Imagawa and colleagues[39] report an 84% rate of curative en bloc resection from 2002 through 2005. The perforation rate was 6%, and each perforation was managed endoscopically. No local recurrences were observed among the 119 curatively resected lesions 1 year after dissection. This technique has even been applied successfully to patients who have undergone insufficient previous endoscopic mucosal resection. Oka and colleagues[40] report successful dissection and resection in 14 of 15 patients who had residual disease after mucosal resection. No recurrences were noted during a mean follow-up period of 18 months. Currently, this technique is being evaluated for the resection of gastric subepithelial tumors from the muscularis propria, including gastrointestinal stromal tumors. Lee and colleagues[41] report the successful excision of 9 in 12 applicable lesions in 11 patients between 2004 and 2006. No patients experienced perforation or hemorrhage.

HIGH-RESOLUTION AND MAGNIFICATION ENDOSCOPY, AND CHROMOENDOSCOPY

To identify lesions amenable for the BARRX Halo system, endoscopic mucosal resection, and endoscopic submucosal dissection treatment modalities, advances had to be made in endoscopic imaging abilities. Conventional endoscopy is characterized by resolution of from 100,000 to 300,000 pixels. Subsequent generations of endoscopic techniques require cameras of 400,000, even 850,000, pixels that are referred to as *high resolution endoscopes*. These endoscopes are equipped with optic zoom composed of movable motor-driven lens. Changing the focus of the lens provides considerable magnification of the observed area, of from 80 to 200 times. It is used in diagnosis of subtle mucosal abnormalities of 1 to 2 mm in diameter to detect early cancerous changes and to direct the precise biopsy of pathological changes.[42,43]

Chromoendoscopy technique uses a locally staining agent applied to the mucous membrane during endoscopy to characterize the changes better. It has become useful in early diagnosis of malignancies and other nonneoplastic conditions. The method is cheap, the coloring agents are widely accessible and nontoxic, and there are no side effects noted if they are used in small, recommended quantities.

Chromoendoscopy became more important when magnifying and high-resolution endoscopy methods were introduced.[44,45] Contrast chromoendoscopy that colors the mucous depressions uses from 1 to 25 mL of 0.1% to 1% solution of indigo carmine (blue pigment), depending on the size of the area examined. The mucosa is examined immediately after the stain has been administered. The method is used to detect early cancers of the esophagus, stomach, and colon, to diagnose Barrett's esophagus, to assess villous atrophy of the intestine, and to detect discrete mucosal loss.[46,47]

Different coloring agents that are absorbed by certain type of cells are used in absorptive staining. Lugol's solution (a dark-brown staining agent) stains glycogen-rich cells of the esophageal epithelium. Following administration, normal, smooth, nonkeratinized esophageal epithelium turns dark brown or green-brown. No change in color suggests abnormal epithelium such as erosive esophagitis, and cancerous metaplastic or dysplastic foci. The inability to differentiate between different conditions requires repeated biopsies of the changed mucosa. Methylene blue 0.2% is a blue staining agent that is actively absorbed by epithelial cells of the small and large intestine. Toluidine blue accumulates in dysplastic and atypical cells with increased DNA proliferation. Toluidine blue stains dysplastic and neoplastic, but not benign, cells dark blue or dark purple-blue. Other staining agents used in absorptive chromoendoscopy are cresyl violet, which diffuses into mucosal depressions, and crystal violet, which stains intestinal metaplastic foci. Absorptive chromoendoscopy is used to diagnose early stages of esophageal cancer and Barrett's esophagus, to locate intestinal metaplastic foci inside the stomach, to identify ectopic gastric mucosa in the duodenum, and to detect colon adenomas and adenocarcinoma.[48] Application of these different stains lengthen the duration of endoscopic procedures considerably, necessitating increased attention to sedation requirements.

DEEP-BALLOON ENTEROSCOPY

Videoenteroscopy is a new endoscopic visualization technique of the small intestine. It was designed by Yamamoto and colleagues in 2001.[49] A typical double-balloon enteroscope is composed of a 200-cm-long endoscope, a 145-cm-long semielastic external tube, and two latex balloons to better fix the endoscope inside the small intestine and for easier penetration. The endoscope can be inserted via the stomach or can be used to approach from the ileocecal valve. The choice of the route depends on the expected localization of the pathology. If the examination of the entire small intestine is required, both routes of insertion should be used after the farthest destination point has been marked with a submucosal marker during the first examination. When the marked point has been reached during subsequent examination using the other route, it implies that the entire length of the small intestine had been examined. Double- and single-balloon techniques, as well as spiral enteroscopy techniques, have been described. The examination of the entire small intestine generally requires more than 2 hours on average, with an increased need for sedation and anesthesiology input. The technique is 80% to 90% effective and failure is most often due to postoperative adhesions.[50] Deep-balloon enteroscopy is recommended in the evaluation of Crohn's disease involving the small bowel, identification of a bleeding source, detection of stenoses and neoplastic changes in the small intestine, and investigation of obscure causes of chronic diarrhea and malabsorption syndromes.[51] Few complications have been described, such as pancreatitis and perforation or microperforation of the small intestine, all of which were treated conservatively.[52,53] In addition to diagnostic possibilities, enteroscopy allows both biopsy of affected areas and endoscopic therapy. The double-balloon enteroscopy method has been the best described and is now considered the "gold standard" in the diagnosis and endoscopic treatment of small intestine diseases. The increased duration of the examination, the sedation requirements, and the use of fluoroscopy may pose some limitations to the procedure.

SUMMARY

A successful population-based colorectal cancer screening requires efficient colonoscopy practices that incorporate high throughput, safety, and patient satisfaction. There are several different modalities of nonanesthesiologist-administered sedation currently available and in development that may fulfill these requirements. Modern-day gastroenterology endoscopic procedures are complex and demand the full attention of the attending gastroenterologist and the complete cooperation of the patient. Many of these procedures will also require the anesthesiologist's knowledge, skills, abilities, and experience to ensure optimal procedure results and good patient outcomes.

REFERENCES

1. Cohen LB, Wecsler JS, Gaetano JN, et al. Endoscopic sedation in the United States: results from a nationwide survey. Am J Gastroenterol 2006;101:967–74.
2. Huang YY, Lee HK, Juan CH, et al. Conscious sedation in gastrointestinal endoscopy. Acta Anaesthesiol Taiwan 2005;43:33–8.
3. Cohen LB, Delegge MH, Aisenberg J, et al. AGA Institute review of endoscopic sedation. Gastroenterology 2007;133:675–701.

4. Byrne MF, Baillie J. Nurse-assisted propofol sedation: the jury is in!. Gastroenterology 2005;129:1781–2.
5. Clarke AC, Chiragakis L, Hillman LC, et al. Sedation for endoscopy: the safe use of propofol by general practitioner sedationists. Med J Aust 2002;176:158–61.
6. Heuss LT, Schnieper P, Drewe J, et al. Safety of propofol for conscious sedation during endoscopic procedures in high-risk patients—a prospective, controlled study. Am J Gastroenterol 2003;98:1751–7.
7. Rex DK, Heuss LT, Walker JA, et al. Trained registered nurses/endoscopy teams can administer propofol safely for endoscopy. Gastroenterology 2005; 129:1384–91.
8. Aisenberg J, Brill JV, Ladabaum U, et al. Sedation for gastrointestinal endoscopy: new practices, new economics. Am J Gastroenterol 2005;100:996–1000.
9. Rex DK. The science and politics of propofol. Am J Gastroenterol 2004;99: 2080–3.
10. Tohda G, Higashi S, Wakahara S, et al. Propofol sedation during endoscopic procedures: safe and effective administration by registered nurses supervised by endoscopists. Endoscopy 2006;38:360–7.
11. Cohen LB, Dubovsky AN, Aisenberg J, et al. Propofol for endoscopic sedation: a protocol for safe and effective administration by the gastroenterologist. Gastrointest Endosc 2003;58:725–32.
12. Cohen LB, Hightower CD, Wood DA, et al. Moderate level sedation during endoscopy: a prospective study using low-dose propofol, meperidine/fentanyl, and midazolam. Gastrointest Endosc 2004;59:795–803.
13. Aisenberg J, Cohen LB, Piorkowski JD Jr. Propofol use under the direction of trained gastroenterologists: an analysis of the medicolegal implications. Am J Gastroenterol 2007;102:707–13.
14. Heuss LT, Drewe J, Schnieper P, et al. Patient-controlled versus nurse-administered sedation with propofol during colonoscopy. A prospective randomized trial. Am J Gastroenterol 2004;99:511–8.
15. Lee DW, Chan AC, Wong SK, et al. The safety, feasibility, and acceptability of patient-controlled sedation for colonoscopy: prospective study. Hong Kong Med J 2004;10:84–8.
16. Egan TD. Target-controlled drug delivery: progress toward an intravenous "vaporizer" and automated anesthetic administration. Anesthesiology 2003;99: 1214–9.
17. Fanti L, Agostoni M, Casati A, et al. Target-controlled propofol infusion during monitored anesthesia in patients undergoing ERCP. Gastrointest Endosc 2004; 60:361–6.
18. Doufas AG, Bakhshandeh M, Bjorksten AR, et al. Induction speed is not a determinant of propofol pharmacodynamics. Anesthesiology 2004;101:1112–21.
19. American Society for Gastrointestinal Endoscopy. Guidelines for training in patient monitoring and sedation and analgesia. Gastrointest Endosc 1998; 48:669–71.
20. Rattner D. Introduction to NOTES White Paper. Surg Endosc 2006;20:185.
21. Rattner D, Kalloo A. ASGE/SAGES Working Group on Natural Orifice Transluminal Endoscopic Surgery. 2005. Surg Endosc 2006;20:329–33.
22. Mintz Y, Horgan S, Cullen J, et al. NOTES: the hybrid technique. J Laparoendosc Adv Surg Tech A 2007;17:402–6.
23. Palanivelu C, Rajan PS, Rangarajan M, et al. Transvaginal endoscopic appendectomy in humans: a unique approach to NOTES—world's first report. Surg Endosc 2008 [Epub ahead of print].

24. Bernhardt J, Gerber B, Schober HC, et al. NOTES—case report of a unidirectional flexible appendectomy. Int J Colorectal Dis 2008;23:547–50.
25. Steele K, Schweitzer MA, Lyn-Sue J, et al. Flexible transgastric peritoneoscopy and liver biopsy: a feasibility study in human beings (with videos). Gastrointest Endosc 2008;68:61–6.
26. Marks JM, Ponsky JL, Pearl JP, et al. PEG "Rescue": a practical NOTES technique. Surg Endosc 2007;21:816–9.
27. Chen YK. Preclinical characterization of the Spyglass peroral cholangiopancreatoscopy system for direct access, visualization, and biopsy. Gastrointest Endosc 2007;65:303–11.
28. Chen YK, Pleskow DK. SpyGlass single-operator peroral cholangiopancreatoscopy system for the diagnosis and therapy of bile-duct disorders: a clinical feasibility study (with video). Gastrointest Endosc 2007;65:832–41.
29. Antillon MR, Tiwari P, Bartalos CR, et al. Taking SpyGlass outside the GI tract lumen in conjunction with EUS to assist in the diagnosis of a pancreatic cystic lesion (with video). Gastrointest Endosc 2008 [Epub ahead of print].
30. Dunkin BJ, Martinez J, Bejarano PA, et al. Thin-layer ablation of human esophageal epithelium using a bipolar radiofrequency balloon device. Surg Endosc 2006;20:125–30.
31. Bergman JJ. Radiofrequency energy ablation of Barrett's esophagus: the best is yet to come! Gastrointest Endosc 2007;65:200–2.
32. Bergman JJ. Endoscopic resection for treatment of mucosal Barrett's cancer: time to swing the pendulum. Gastrointest Endosc 2007;65:11–3.
33. Deprez PH, Aouattah T, Piessevaux H. Endoscopic removal or ablation of oesophageal and gastric superficial tumours. Acta Gastroenterol Belg 2006;69:304–11.
34. Ross AS, Noffsinger A, Waxman I. Narrow band imaging directed EMR for Barrett's esophagus with high-grade dysplasia. Gastrointest Endosc 2007;65:166–9.
35. Ell C, May A, Pech O, et al. Curative endoscopic resection of early esophageal adenocarcinomas (Barrett's cancer). Gastrointest Endosc 2007;65:3–10.
36. Seewald S, Ang TL, Omar S, et al. Endoscopic mucosal resection of early esophageal squamous cell cancer using the Duette mucosectomy kit. Endoscopy 2006;38:1029–31.
37. Jaquet Y, Pilloud R, Grosjean P, et al. Extended endoscopic mucosal resection in the esophagus and hypopharynx: a new rigid device. Eur Arch Otorhinolaryngol 2007;264:57–62.
38. Gotoda T, Yamamoto H, Soetikno RM. Endoscopic submucosal dissection of early gastric cancer. J Gastroenterol 2006;41:929–42.
39. Imagawa A, Okada H, Kawahara Y, et al. Endoscopic submucosal dissection for early gastric cancer: results and degrees of technical difficulty as well as success. Endoscopy 2006;38:987–90.
40. Oka S, Tanaka S, Kaneko I, et al. Endoscopic submucosal dissection for residual/local recurrence of early gastric cancer after endoscopic mucosal resection. Endoscopy 2006;38:996–1000.
41. Lee II, Lin PY, Tung SY, et al. Endoscopic submucosal dissection for the treatment of intraluminal gastric subepithelial tumors originating from the muscularis propria layer. Endoscopy 2006;38:1024–8.
42. Nelson DB, Block KP, Bosco JJ, et al. High resolution and high-magnification endoscopy: September 2000. Gastrointest Endosc 2000;52:864–6.
43. Skrzypek T, Valverde Piedra JL, Skrzypek H, et al. Light and scanning electron microscopy evaluation of the postnatal small intestinal mucosa development in pigs. J Physiol Pharmacol 2005;56(Suppl 3):71–87.

44. Acosta MM, Boyce HW Jr. Chromoendoscopy—where is it useful? J Clin Gastroenterol 1998;27:13–20.
45. Fennerty MB. Tissue staining (chromoscopy) of the gastrointestinal tract. Can J Gastroenterol 1999;13:423–9.
46. Kiesslich R, Mergener K, Naumann C, et al. Value of chromoendoscopy and magnification endoscopy in the evaluation of duodenal abnormalities: a prospective, randomized comparison. Endoscopy 2003;35:559–63.
47. Stevens PD, Lightdale CJ, Green PH, et al. Combined magnification endoscopy with chromoendoscopy for the evaluation of Barrett's esophagus. Gastrointest Endosc 1994;40:747–9.
48. Tabuchi M, Sueoka N, Fujimori T. Videoendoscopy with vital double dye staining (crystal violet and methylene blue) for detection of a minute focus of early stage adenocarcinoma in Barrett's esophagus: a case report. Gastrointest Endosc 2001;54:385–8.
49. Yamamoto H, Sekine Y, Sato Y, et al. Total enteroscopy with a nonsurgical steerable double-balloon method. Gastrointest Endosc 2001;53:216–20.
50. May A, Nachbar L, Schneider M, et al. Push-and-pull enteroscopy using the double-balloon technique: method of assessing depth of insertion and training of the enteroscopy technique using the Erlangen Endo-Trainer. Endoscopy 2005;37:66–70.
51. May A, Nachbar L, Ell C. Double-balloon enteroscopy (push-and-pull enteroscopy) of the small bowel: feasibility and diagnostic and therapeutic yield in patients with suspected small bowel disease. Gastrointest Endosc 2005;62:62–70.
52. Mensink PB, Haringsma J, Kucharzik T, et al. Complications of double balloon enteroscopy: a multicenter survey. Endoscopy 2007;39:613–5.
53. Yamamoto H, Kita H, Sunada K, et al. Clinical outcomes of double-balloon endoscopy for the diagnosis and treatment of small-intestinal diseases. Clin Gastroenterol Hepatol 2004;2:1010–6.

Anesthesia for Gastrointestinal Endoscopic Procedures

Daniel T. Goulson, MD*, Regina Y. Fragneto, MD

KEYWORDS

- Anesthesia • Sedation
- Esophagogastroduodenoscopy • Colonoscopy
- Endoscopic retrograde cholangiopancreatography
- Endoscopic ultrasonography

The provision of sedation and analgesia always has been a critical component of performing endoscopic procedures on the gastrointestinal (GI) tract. The procedures create some pain and discomfort and are associated with anxiety for the patient. Of course, comfort is paramount, but patient cooperation also is critical to the success of the examination. In the early days of endoscopy, it was routine practice for the sedation and analgesia to be provided by the endoscopist, who ordered a benzodiazepine, such as diazepam, and an opioid, such as meperidine, that were administered by a nurse. Monitoring was provided by periodic visual observation by the physician and/or the nurse. The administration of supplemental oxygen was inconsistent.

In the current environment, things are changing. The demand for endoscopy, especially screening colonoscopies, has increased dramatically. More stimulating and complex procedures that can be accomplished with the endoscope are emerging. New medications for sedation and analgesia are either under investigation or already are on the market. Standards for monitoring and criteria for discharge are improving.

Because of these changes, anesthesiologists have become involved in the care of many of these patients.[1] In some situations, endoscopists may not want to divide their attention between performing the procedure and maintaining the sedation. In other situations, there may be a need for more sophisticated medications that require the expertise of an anesthesiologist. Occasionally, the need for sedation is escalated, sometimes to the point of requiring general anesthesia, because of the complexity of the procedure. Last, these procedures also are becoming common in children, whose cooperation may be gained only with the administration of general anesthesia.

Department of Anesthesiology, University of Kentucky College of Medicine, 800 Rose Street, Lexington, KY 40536, USA
* Corresponding author.
E-mail address: dgoul0@email.uky.edu (D.T. Goulson).

Anesthesiology Clin 27 (2009) 71–85
doi:10.1016/j.anclin.2008.10.004
1932-2275/08/$ – see front matter © 2009 Elsevier Inc. All rights reserved.

anesthesiology.theclinics.com

The provision of anesthesia or sedation for endoscopy is associated with issues that are different from care during surgical cases. Some of those areas of difference relate to the location in which the care is provided, relationships with the endoscopists, relationships with payors, varying levels of patient preparation, the use of different medications, and the management of complications in an out-of-operating-room environment. This article covers all of these areas.

VENUES

Historically, GI endoscopy was performed in a hospital setting. A recent survey of members of the American College of Gastroenterology shows this still is true most of the time. The ambulatory surgery center (ASC) now is becoming the preferred location for these procedures,[2] however, and approximately 35.8% of endoscopists consider an ASC as their primary location for performance of endoscopy.[1] There seem to be significant regional differences in where endoscopies are done. For example, office endoscopy accounted for 19.8% of procedures in the Mid-Atlantic region but only 0.4% in the Northeast in the 2004 survey.[1] Some of these differences are related to reimbursement issues,[3] and some are related to local customs and practices.

From the perspective of the anesthesiologist, the venue is important for several reasons. The most important is the capability for patient monitoring and resuscitation that is available in a particular location. Secondary considerations involve the scheduling and availability of anesthesia personnel, if requested for assistance in the sedation. Most anesthesiologists believe that an operating room provides the most flexibility for caring for medically challenging patients. Endoscopy equipment is relatively portable, compared with the equipment for other nonsurgical procedures in which anesthesiologists are involved (eg, CT scanning). This portability makes it possible for endoscopy cases to be treated in an operating room even if that location is not the endoscopist's preference.

SEDATION VERSUS GENERAL ANESTHESIA

In the survey mentioned previously, gastroenterologists in the United States reported that sedation is provided for 98% to 99% of esophagogastroduodenoscopies (EGDs) and colonoscopies.[1] It seems likely that this nearly universal use of sedation also is the practice for other procedures performed in the GI suite, such as endoscopic retrograde cholangiopancreatography (ERCP) and endoscopic ultrasonography (EUS). Most patients received sedation under the supervision of the gastroenterologist; the survey reported that anesthesia care providers (both anesthesiologists and certified registered nurse anesthetists) were responsible for providing sedation in approximately 28% of cases. Of note, the use of anesthesia personnel varies widely among geographic areas. Fewer than 10% of patients undergoing procedures in the Northeast, Midwest, and Southwest regions have an anesthesia care provider involved in their care, but 17% of patients in the South and more than one third of patients in the Mid-Atlantic area have anesthesia professionals responsible for administering their sedation. Some of these regional differences may be economically driven and are discussed later in this article. Although are no data are available to describe what patient characteristics prompt the GI physician to use anesthesia professionals, the experience of most anesthesiologists is that they are asked to care primarily for pediatric patients, patients who have a history of being difficult to sedate, and patients who have life-threatening medical conditions.

When anesthetizing patients in the GI suite, an anesthesiologist first must decide what level of sedation or anesthesia is required. Many factors play a role in this decision-making process. The patient's medical status, including whether the patient is at risk for aspiration and requires protection of the airway with an endotracheal tube, is an essential factor to consider. The complexity of the GI procedure, the patient position required to perform the procedure, and the proximity of the anesthesia care provider to the patient's airway during the procedure also must be considered when developing an anesthetic plan. Other factors that often are used in this decision-making process include a patient's history of failed sedation by non-anesthesia health care providers, substance abuse, or mental illness.

Relatively healthy patients who are undergoing simpler procedures, such as EGD or colonoscopy, often tolerate the procedure well with moderate sedation. At many institutions these patients are sedated without the involvement of anesthesia personnel. A significant number of GI facilities, however, do use anesthesia care providers for nearly all sedation procedures, and anesthesiologists can expect to provide moderate sedation to the most of their patients in such a practice setting. In most GI units, however, anesthesia professionals usually are involved only for more complex patients or procedures. These situations often require deep sedation or general anesthesia to achieve adequate patient comfort, cooperation, and optimal operating conditions for the GI physician.

One challenge for both gastroenterologists and anesthesiologists is to predict before the procedure which patients will require deep sedation or general anesthesia not because of the patient's medical condition or the complexity of the procedure but to provide sufficient patient cooperation and comfort. Data to determine patient factors that could assist in identifying patients who may be difficult to sedate do not seem to be available and could be the focus of future study. In areas outside North America, many patients undergo simple GI procedures, such as EGD, without any sedation. There are data from Europe identifying factors that predict poor patient tolerance of an unsedated EGD, and these same patient characteristics also might predict patients who will require deeper levels of sedation or general anesthesia for a successful procedure in practice settings where sedation is used for all patients. Both apprehension about the procedure, as rated by the patient, and high levels of anxiety, as measured by administering the state trait anxiety inventory before the procedure, were associated with poor patient tolerance.[4]

OTHER PRACTICAL ISSUES
Scheduling

Facility scheduling for endoscopic procedures shares many characteristics with scheduling for surgical procedures. One consideration is the availability of multiple resources, including the endoscopist, nursing personnel, endoscopy equipment, and a physical location for the procedure. Some gastroenterologists favor an open-access model of scheduling[5] in which patients are referred from other physicians and there is no preprocedure office visit. This method does present challenges in assuring that the proper procedure is indicated and that the patient is prepared adequately.

If the gastroenterology practice uses an anesthesiologist to provide sedation for only selected cases, the matter of scheduling becomes even more complicated. The availability of an anesthesiologist then must be considered as an additional resource that must be scheduled. Cases requiring the service of an anesthesiologist should be grouped together when possible to increase the likelihood of financial viability for that provider. If the volume of sedation cases is large enough, an anesthesiologist may dedicate the entire day to the endoscopy facility. Otherwise, the anesthesiologist probably will spend part of the day providing sedation for endoscopies and part of the day providing anesthesia in another location.

Preprocedure Evaluation

If the expectation is that the anesthesiologist will provide deep sedation or general anesthesia for a patient, the principles of pre-anesthetic evaluation that apply to surgical cases should apply to these endoscopic cases also. This evaluation requires a significant amount of communication between the anesthesiologist and the gastroenterologist about the patients in question. If there is a well-defined process, the patient must follow the same steps for evaluation. Depending on the patient's condition, these steps could include laboratory testing and EKG and echocardiographic evaluations. If processes for routine performance of a pre-anesthetic evaluation are not in place, the anesthesiologist must ensure that the gastroenterologist understands the expectations regarding pre-anesthetic evaluation.

The pre-anesthetic evaluation has become one of the challenges of providing anesthesia for these cases. Often the patient arrives in the facility for monitored anesthesia care or general anesthesia poorly prepared for an anesthetic. This situation results in frustration for everyone involved.

One area of particular concern is management of antiplatelet medications, especially when patients have had recent placement of a drug-eluting stent. This concern is pertinent in procedures in which there is a chance for bleeding, such as banding of esophageal varices or ERCP with sphincterotomy. As with surgical cases, the decision of whether to withhold these medications is complex and must be made in collaboration with the cardiologist, gastroenterologist, and anesthesiologist. One approach that has been advocated when patients are taking anticoagulants[6] is to perform an initial diagnostic endoscopy for visualization only while the still patient is following the usual anticoagulant regimen. Once the results of that endoscopy are known, an informed decision can be made about managing anticoagulation if a therapeutic endoscopy is needed. It is reassuring that a small case-control study of ERCP with sphincterotomy suggested that the risk of clinically significant bleeding is not increased in patients who have been taking antiplatelet medications within 10 days of the procedure.[7]

Reimbursement for Sedation and Analgesia

In the traditional model in which the gastroenterologist administers sedation, payors typically do not provide separate reimbursement for the sedation. As anesthesiologists have begun to provide this service, separate claims are being submitted for the sedation. Estimates are that charges to Medicare for anesthesia for colonoscopy increased by 86% between 2001 and 2003, to $80,000,000.[3] In response to that rapid rise, payment for anesthesia for endoscopy has been scrutinized. Most payors distinguish between high-risk and average-risk cases. In general, they have allowed charges for anesthesia in high-risk patients. Payment policies for average-risk patients are evolving, however, and there are differences among Medicare contractors. Consequently, regional differences in practice have developed that seem to be influenced by reimbursement patterns. For example, the growth in charges by anesthesiologists to Empire Medicare Services[3] in the metropolitan New York area is far steeper than the national growth rate, presumably in part because at this Medicare contractor's policies allow reimbursement.

MEDICATIONS FOR SEDATION AND ANALGESIA

The most widely used combination for sedation for GI endoscopy is a benzodiazepine, such as midazolam, and an opioid, such as meperidine or fentanyl,[8] but several other medications have been explored in the quest for ease of titration, rapid recovery, and minimization of untoward side effects.[9]

Propofol

Propofol is an agent that typically has been used for general anesthesia, but in sub-hypnotic doses it can produce moderate levels of sedation. Its therapeutic window is very narrow, making it easy to move from the level of moderate sedation into deep sedation or general anesthesia. Therefore the Food and Drug Administration (FDA) product label currently states that propofol "should only be administered by persons trained in the administration of general anesthesia," which also would give them the ability to rescue a patient from unintended levels of deep sedation.[10] This practice also is consistent with the Joint Commission for the Accreditation of Health Care Organization's current approach to sedation. Their standards state that practitioners providing sedation should be able to rescue patients who slip into a deeper-than-desired level of sedation.[11] Specifically, persons providing moderate sedation should be qualified to rescue patients from deep sedation and be competent to manage a compromised airway and provide adequate oxygenation and ventilation.

The drive to use propofol as an adjunct to endoscopy goes hand-in-hand with the increased demand for these procedures. Because the practice of endoscopists has become busier, there are increased needs for efficiency.[9] In the past, prolonged recovery and relatively long discharge times resulted in a loss of efficiency. Because propofol has a fast onset and allows rapid recovery, gastroenterologists have become interested in using it for their procedures. The restrictions mentioned previously, however, suggest that an anesthesiologist should be involved in the sedation.

These governmental restrictions are not as clear-cut in other countries. Quoting a worldwide experience with gastroenterologist-directed administration of propofol for procedural sedation in 200,000 patient encounters with no mortalities, several gastroenterology-related professional societies have questioned the medical necessity of restricting its use to anesthesiologists.[8] In 2005, the American College of Gastroenterology petitioned the United States FDA to remove the section of the warning label pertaining to administration by individuals trained in general anesthesia.[12]

In response to the current political and regulatory environment and in combination with escalating costs associated with administering propofol by an anesthesiologist in the United States, several alternative models of administration have emerged.[13] One alternative is nurse-administered propofol sedation. In this model, propofol is administered by registered nurses under a strict protocol and under the supervision of the endoscopist.[14] There are several studies of this model in the literature, covering more than 200,000 administrations. Questions still remain about the true incidences of airway complications[13] and need for airway interventions. Debate also continues about whether this model obviates the need for the endoscopist to have skills in deep sedation and airway rescue.

Another alternative model for propofol administration is patient-controlled sedation. The theoretic advantage of patient-controlled sedation is that it allows the patient to match his or her sedation needs to the discomfort of the procedure while avoiding the effects of oversedation.[13] This model is discussed further later in this article.

Fospropofol

Fospropofol is a water-soluble prodrug of propofol that currently is being evaluated as a sedative agent for diagnostic and therapeutic procedures.[15] It is hydrolyzed rapidly to release propofol. Following intravenous (IV) administration, the plasma concentration profile of fospropofol-derived propofol is characterized by a smooth and predictable rise and decline instead of the rapid spike observed following administration of the lipid-emulsion formulation of propofol. The elimination kinetics of propofol is similar, whether it was derived from fospropofol or not.

One dose-ranging study appears in the literature. Cohen[15] studied 127 patients receiving either midazolam or one of four different doses of fospropofol for sedation for elective colonoscopy. The investigators examined rates of sedation success, time to sedation, requirements for alternative sedative medication, requirements for assisted ventilation, supplemental doses of sedative, time to discharge, and satisfaction of the physician with the sedation. Only one patient required any kind of airway intervention, and that was verbal stimulation to address hypoxemia. The investigators concluded that the 6.5-mg/kg dose provided the ideal balance of efficacy and safety.

The medication is currently under phase III trials and has not yet been approved for use in the United States. Interestingly, the American Society of Anesthesiologists has submitted formal comments to the FDA requesting that the fospropofol label contain restrictions similar to those for propofol,[16] because they believe that this drug also will be able to produce a state of general anesthesia in patients.

Dexmedetomidine

Dexmedetomidine is another relatively new agent that has been considered for sedation for endoscopy. It is a highly selective α_2-adrenoreceptor agonist with sedative and analgesic effects[17] that was approved in 1999 by the FDA for sedation in patients in ICUs.[18] One significant reported advantage is that patients can be sedated but are able to be roused to full consciousness easily.[19]

Only a handful of studies have examined this agent specifically in the setting of endoscopy. Demiraran and colleagues[20] compared dexmedetomidine and midazolam as the sedative agent for EGD. No opioids were given in this small study of 50 patients that was performed in Turkey. The investigators concluded that dexmedetomidine and midazolam have similar efficacy and safety profiles.

Another study from Poland examined dexmedetomidine in comparison with meperidine or fentanyl as a single agent for sedation for colonoscopy. The investigators found that patients in the dexmedetomidine group required significant supplemental fentanyl and had a high risk of bradycardia and hypotension. They concluded was that dexmedetomidine is not a suitable agent for sedation.[21]

Ketamine

Ketamine has been examined both as a sole agent and in combination with other medications in adults and children. Most references in the literature relate to its use in children. Gilger and colleagues[22] retrospectively examined 402 procedures in which various combinations of midazolam, meperidine, and ketamine were used. They found that the midazolam/ketamine combination had the lowest rate of complications and a rate of adequate sedation equivalent to that of the other combinations. Intramuscular ketamine also has been studied as a sole agent for sedation in pediatric endoscopy but was found to have a high failure rate in a small study.[23] Kirberg and colleagues[24] have described their experience with ketamine in both pediatric endoscopy and adult endoscopy and have found it to be an effective agent. In advanced endoscopic procedures in adults, such as ERCP and EUS, ketamine is a useful adjunct to more traditional sedation agents and helps produce acceptable procedural conditions.[25]

Benzodiazepines

Benzodiazepines have long been an integral part of the sedation regimen for GI endoscopy. The early preparations of IV benzodiazepines were lipid soluble, creating issues with administration. During that time, diazepam was the medication in this class most frequently used for endoscopy. Once water-soluble midazolam became available in the late 1980s, it quickly gained favor.[26] Today, midazolam is strongly favored over diazepam.[1]

Opioids

The second part of the conventional sedation combination is an opioid. Twenty years ago, meperidine was a mainstay.[26] Today, meperidine and fentanyl are used about equally.[1] Some practitioners also have begun to use other fast-acting opioids such as remifentanil,[27] although usually not as a single agent.

SEDATION/ANESTHESIA FOR SPECIFIC PROCEDURES

GI endoscopic procedures vary significantly in their complexity and the degree of patient stimulation and pain that occur. Therefore, the optimal sedation or anesthetic techniques for various procedures for various procedures differ.

Esophagogastroduodenoscopy

Adequate sedation for EGD can be achieved in most patients with a combination of an IV benzodiazepine and opioid, but most anesthesiologists use IV propofol for EGD sedations. When surveyed, gastroenterologists have reported greater satisfaction with propofol than with the conventional sedation technique of benzodiazepine and an opioid. In fact, the median satisfaction score for propofol was 10 on a 10-point scale in which 10 was defined as best.[1] Moderate and deep sedation as well as general anesthesia can be achieved with propofol. Patients who have a history of substance abuse or of being difficult to sedate usually require deep sedation or general anesthesia for an EGD procedure. Even when moderate sedation is the intended goal for the procedure, however, deep sedation often is achieved. In one study, 60% of patients undergoing EGD reached a level of deep sedation despite a preprocedure plan for moderate sedation.[28]

Another factor to consider when choosing between sedation and general anesthesia for EGD is whether endotracheal intubation is needed. The indication for performing EGD, such as persistent vomiting or severe gastroesophageal reflux disease, may dictate protection of the airway with an endotracheal tube. In other patients, such as those who are obese or who have obstructive sleep apnea, significant airway obstruction during deep sedation may necessitate endotracheal intubation. Patients who do undergo endotracheal intubation usually require a level of general anesthesia to tolerate adequately both the endoscopic procedure and the presence of the endotracheal tube.

A unique anesthetic technique for EGD that has been reported is general anesthesia via a ProSeal laryngeal mask airway (LMA).[29] The drain tube of this specialized LMA can serve as a conduit to guide the gastroscope into the stomach, thus possibly improving the ease of the endoscopic procedure for the gastroenterologist. In the recent study that described this technique, the anesthesia and endoscopy times were significantly shorter in the group of patients randomly assigned to the use of the ProSeal LMA than in patients who received the same anesthetic drugs but whose airways were managed with chin lift/jaw thrust as needed and oxygen via nasal cannula. In addition, the mean oxygen saturation was higher and fewer episodes of arterial oxyhemoglobin saturation (SpO_2) less than 90% occurred in the ProSeal group than in the nasal cannula group.

An adjunct to sedation for EGD that often is overlooked but should be considered by anesthesiologists is topical pharyngeal anesthesia. Although some studies have reported no added benefit from topical anesthesia in sedated patients,[30] other individual studies[31] as well as a meta-analysis[32] have reported that ease of endoscopy is improved in patients who receive topical pharyngeal anesthesia in addition to sedation. In the United States, commercially available local anesthetic sprays, including Cetacaine and Hurricane sprays, are used most commonly to provide pharyngeal anesthesia. These sprays contain benzocaine, which has been associated with the development of methemoglobinemia.[33] Another option for topical anesthesia that could avoid the risk of methemoglobinemia is use of a lidocaine lollipop. Investigators at an institution in Lebanon found this technique very effective. In fact, only one third of patients who received the lollipop required IV sedation for EGD, whereas nearly 100% of the patients who did not receive topical anesthesia required sedation.[34]

Colonoscopy

Like EGD, adequate sedation for colonoscopy can be achieved with a combination of benzodiazepine and an opioid in most patients. One study found that when moderate sedation was planned, deep sedation was less likely to be achieved during colonoscopy than during EGD, ERCP, or EUS.[28] This difference may be explained by the apparently less stimulating nature of colonoscopy compared with the other procedures. When anesthesia professionals provide sedation for colonoscopy, however, they usually use propofol and often plan to attain a level of deep sedation or general anesthesia. In fact, it seems likely that even when gastroenterologists are responsible for the sedation during colonoscopy, they and their patients actually prefer to achieve at least deep sedation rather than moderate sedation. In a study of nurse-administered propofol sedation that was performed under the supervision of the GI physician, the mean bispectral index score was 59, indicating a state of general anesthesia.[35]

Several sedation or anesthesia techniques for colonoscopy have been studied. Remifentanil is a very short-acting opioid that may offer advantages for patients undergoing outpatient colonoscopy. Moerman and colleagues[36] compared IV remifentanil versus IV propofol. They found that measures of early recovery, such as spontaneous eye opening and following commands, occurred sooner in the patients who received remifentanil. Recovery of cognitive function also was faster with remifentanil than with propofol. Respiratory depression occurred more frequently in the remifentanil group, however, and patient satisfaction was lower in this group than in the propofol group. In another study that compared remifentanil and propofol, postprocedure nausea and vomiting was a significant problem with remifentanil sedation.[37] General anesthesia using an inhalational technique of sevoflurane/nitrous oxide has been compared with total IV anesthesia (TIVA) using propofol/fentanyl/midazolam for colonoscopy. Patients who received the inhalational anesthetic were less sedated 20 minutes after the procedure than patients who received TIVA. A greater degree of psychomotor impairment that lasted longer also was reported in the TIVA group.[38]

The use of propofol alone to achieve deep sedation has been compared with lower doses of propofol in combination with fentanyl and/or midazolam titrated to moderate sedation. Patients who received the combination therapy were discharged more quickly than patients who received only propofol with no differences found between the groups in satisfaction scores, vital signs, or oxygen saturation.[39]

Patient-controlled sedation with propofol is a new technique that seems to be effective for sedation during colonoscopy. A prospective, randomized study in France compared patient-controlled sedation with anesthesiologist-administered propofol. Patients in the patient-controlled group self-administered 20-mg boluses of propofol as needed with a lock-out time of 1 minute. Patients in the anesthesiologist-controlled group received a continuous infusion of propofol that was titrated to effect. Success of the colonoscopy, which was defined by reaching the cecum, and technical ease of the procedure as rated by the gastroenterologist did not differ between the groups. In addition, patient satisfaction was similar between the groups. Several advantages were reported for patient-controlled propofol administration compared with administration by an anesthesiologist. Depth of sedation was less in the patient-controlled group, and fewer episodes of SpO_2 less than 94% were reported. Time to discharge also was shorter with patient-controlled sedation. The most striking difference reported was the mean total dose of propofol administered: 60 mg in the patient-controlled group versus 248 mg in the physician-administered group.[40] It is quite probable that patient-controlled sedation may become a preferred method of sedation for colonoscopy in the future.

Endoscopic Retrograde Cholangiopancreatography

Patients undergoing ERCP often are more severely ill than patients undergoing EGD or colonoscopy. Common presenting diagnoses include pancreatitis, pancreatic cancer, and cholangitis. The serious medical conditions of these patients may account in part for the high risk of cardiopulmonary complications associated with ERCP. In one study of patients cared for by anesthesia care providers, approximately 25% of patients age 65 years or older developed new electrocardiographic changes during or after ERCP, and 11% of patients in that age group had elevated cardiac troponin levels after the procedure.[41] Relatively complex therapeutic procedures that are of longer duration than EGD or colonoscopy, such as biliary sphincterotomy, removal of bile duct stones, and placement of biliary stents, frequently are undertaken during the ERCP. Patient immobility is an important factor in the successful completion of these technically challenging procedures. Most endoscopists perform ERCP in the prone position. Finally, some of these patients require chronic opioid therapy because of their underlying biliary disease. Therefore, management of patients presenting for ERCP often is more challenging for the anesthesiologist than providing anesthesia for EGD or colonoscopy.

Despite these challenges, some anesthesiologists successfully provide moderate or deep sedation for ERCP. Propofol usually is the preferred sedative drug. One study compared sedation with midazolam or propofol. The procedure was completed successfully more often in patients receiving propofol (97.5%, versus 80% for midazolam), and recovery time was significantly shorter.[42] Anesthesiologists also have provided successful sedation for ERCP by using a target-controlled infusion of propofol and titrating to a target concentration of 2 to 5 µg/mL.[43]

Several of these issues encountered with ERCP have led many anesthesiologists to prefer general anesthesia for this procedure. There are data that support this clinical approach. In one retrospective study of more than 1000 patients, the ERCP failure rate with moderate sedation was double that with general anesthesia (14% versus 7%), with most failures resulting from inadequate sedation.[44] It also has been reported that complication rates associated with therapeutic interventions during ERCP may be significantly lower when general anesthesia is used, perhaps because the absence of patient movement makes the procedure technically less difficult.[45]

When general anesthesia is administered for ERCP, the airway often is protected by endotracheal intubation because of the prone position required during the procedure and because of the presence of risk factors for aspiration in some patients. Investigators, however, have used the LMA successfully for ERCP performed under general anesthesia, in some cases even placing the LMA while the patient was in the prone position. They reported that the endoscope was advanced without difficulty, and time to removal of the airway device was shorter than in patients who underwent endotracheal intubation.[46]

Endoscopic Ultrasonography

Like ERCP, EUS is a more complex procedure than EGD or colonoscopy. It is used for diagnosing and staging GI and pancreatic tumors. Needle-aspiration biopsies often are performed that require examination by a pathologist to determine the adequacy of the sample before the procedure can be completed. Therefore, EUS procedures may be relatively long in duration. In addition, the specialized ultrasound-containing endoscope is significantly larger than a standard endoscope, and insertion causes more patient discomfort than experienced during EGD. As a result, adequate sedation for the procedure is more likely to require deep sedation or general anesthesia.

Some patients satisfactorily tolerate an EUS procedure with a combination of benzodiazepine and an opioid. Titration to an adequate level of sedation while avoiding airway obstruction and hypoxemia may be more problematic during EUS than during EGD or colonoscopy, however. As a result, alternative sedation techniques have been investigated. In one study, preprocedure sedation with moderate doses of benzodiazepine and an opioid were supplemented as needed during the EUS with either ketamine or additional doses of the benzodiazepine and opioid. Improved sedation (as measured by patient comfort and degree of sedation-related technical difficulty) and faster recovery were achieved with ketamine. In addition, approximately one third of patients who were assigned randomly to the benzodiazepine/opioid arm of the study had to cross over to ketamine to achieve an adequate level of sedation to complete the EUS successfully.[25]

Propofol, of course, is another preferred anesthetic drug for EUS. A propofol infusion controlled manually by the anesthesiologist is used most commonly, but other techniques, including a target-controlled propofol infusion, have been used successfully for sedation during EUS. Because preprocedure anxiolysis is beneficial in some patients, one group of investigators studied the effect of administering a dose of midazolam before initiating the target-controlled infusion. Administration of midazolam did not reduce significantly the amount of propofol required during the EUS, but it also did not delay the time to discharge readiness.[47] Patient-controlled sedation with propofol and fentanyl, using 4.25-mg boluses of propofol and 3.75-μg boluses of fentanyl without a lock-out time, also has provided sedation successfully during EUS.[48]

Pediatric Procedures

Most pediatric patients require deep sedation or general anesthesia to tolerate GI endoscopic procedures. Therefore, anesthesiologists are more likely to participate in pediatric procedures than in adult procedures. At many institutions, anesthesia care providers administer the sedation or anesthesia for all or most pediatric endoscopies. Many of the anesthetic principles and drugs used in caring for adult GI patients are pertinent in the pediatric population, but there are additional challenges. Typically, pediatric patients require larger per-weight doses of the sedative medications than adults. One group of investigators determined the median effective concentration of propofol required for EGD in children. It was significantly higher (3.55 μg/mL) than the usual concentration required in adults undergoing this procedure.[49]

Other challenges encountered when caring for children in the GI suite that are unique to the pediatric population are distress caused by the insertion of an IV catheter and by separation from parents. When young children are anesthetized in the operating room, IV catheters usually are placed after mask induction with a volatile anesthetic agent. At many GI facilities, it is not practical to have an anesthesia machine available, and IV drugs are used to provide both sedation and general anesthesia. Insertion of the IV catheter often is the most difficult part of the sedation procedure for everyone involved (patient, parents, and practitioner). Techniques that can facilitate IV placement as well as separation from the parents are invaluable. In one study, pre-procedure administration of oral midazolam was more effective in improving both concerns than the use of IV propofol only. The researchers also found that administration of oral midazolam significantly decreased the dose of propofol required during endoscopy. Recovery time was significantly longer in patients who received midazolam, but longer recovery time seems a small price to pay to make the procedure less traumatic for both child and parents, especially because the mean recovery time still was only 26 minutes.[50]

MANAGING COMPLICATIONS

One prospective cohort study has reported on cardiopulmonary complications that occurred during nearly 12,000 colonoscopies or EGDs in which patients received monitored anesthesia care with propofol. The overall rate of complications was 0.86% for colonoscopy and 1.01% for EGD. The rate of serious adverse events was much lower, however: 13 of 8129 colonoscopies and 6 of 3762 EGDs. Of interest, the rate of complications was lower for both procedures when an anesthesia practitioner, rather than a gastroenterologist, provided sedation.[51] There are few other data available about sedation or anesthesia-related complications associated with GI endoscopy when sedation was provided by an anesthesiologist.

Despite the limited data, anesthesiologists should anticipate that anesthetic complications will occur occasionally. The principles for management of these complications do not differ from management in the operating room, but anesthesia practitioners also must realize that the resources available for handling these problems in the operating room suite may not be as readily accessible in the endoscopy suite. Support personnel in the operating room may be comfortable assisting anesthesiologists during acute cardiopulmonary events, but nursing staff in the GI suite have more limited exposure to such events and may not be able to provide the same level of assistance. Necessary equipment, such as that needed for advanced airway techniques, may not be available immediately. Before providing anesthesia services in the endoscopy unit, the anesthesiologist should anticipate, based on the patient's medical condition, what equipment might be needed and have it present in the GI suite. The anesthesiologist also should have a plan for obtaining additional assistance in the event of a serious adverse event. Many of these endoscopy procedures can be performed in an operating room. In certain high-risk patients, it is appropriate to request that the anesthetizing location be moved to the operating room where serious anesthesia-related complications can be managed more efficiently and effectively.

POSTANESTHESIA RECOVERY

At facilities where most endoscopy procedures are performed with gastroenterologist-administered moderate sedation, the anesthesiologist must understand fully the capabilities of the nursing staff responsible for monitoring patients during the recovery period. These units sometimes are equipped only to provide nursing care at the level necessary for monitoring patients who have received moderate sedation. It is essential that patients who have received deep sedation or general anesthesia for their endoscopy procedures receive the same level of nursing care they would in the post-anesthesia care unit (PACU) of the institution's surgical suite. In fact, regulatory organizations such as the Joint Commission for Accreditation of Health Care Organizations require that equivalent postanesthesia care be delivered in all locations within the health care facility. Information such as the type of training the recovery nurses in the endoscopy suite have received (eg, is the training equivalent to that required of nurses who work in the surgical postanesthesia care unit?) and whether the same patient/nurse staffing ratio used in the surgical PACU can be achieved in the GI suite must be determined when deciding on the appropriate location for recovery of these patients. If adequate nursing care is available, it is preferable for the postanesthesia recovery to occur in the endoscopy suite to avoid transportation of the patient to another location in the immediate postprocedure period. If the anesthesia care provider does not feel comfortable with the level of care available in the GI suite, however, arrangements to transfer the patient to the surgical suite's PACU should be made. Even when satisfactory recovery room care is available in the endoscopy suite, it may be advisable to monitor patients who are at especially high risk for developing anesthesia-related complications in a unit such as the surgical suite's PACU, where these complications are encountered and managed on a frequent basis.

Discharge criteria should be the same as those used for patients who receive anesthesia or sedation in the operating room. Recovery nurses need to understand fully the criteria and know how to contact anesthesia personnel for assistance during the recovery period. Postanesthesia management of patients who have obstructive sleep apnea may be especially challenging. Based on the guidelines published by the American Society of Anesthesiologists,[52] it should be expected that prolonged recovery times may be required for these patients. If logistical or staffing issues do not allow extended monitoring of these patients, arrangements for postanesthesia recovery in another location will be necessary.

REFERENCES

1. Cohen LB, Wecsler JS, Gaetano JN, et al. Endoscopic sedation in the United States: results from a nationwide survey. Am J Gastroenterol 2006;101:967–74.
2. Frakes JT. Outpatient endoscopy. The case for the ambulatory surgery center. Gastrointest Endosc Clin N Am 2002;12:215–27.
3. Aisenberg J, Brill JV, Ladabaum U, et al. Sedation for gastrointestinal endoscopy: new practices, new economics. Am J Gastroenterol 2005;100:996–1000.
4. Campo R, Brullet E, Montserrat A, et al. Identification of factors that influence tolerance of upper gastrointestinal endoscopy. Eur J Gastroenterol Hepatol 1999;11:201–4.
5. Pike IM. Open-access endoscopy. Gastrointest Endosc Clin N Am 2006;16:709–17.
6. Mathew A, Riley TR 3rd, Young M, et al. Cost-saving approach to patients on long-term anticoagulation who need endoscopy: a decision analysis. Am J Gastroenterol 2003;98:1766–76.
7. Hussain N, Alsulaiman R, Burtin P, et al. The safety of endoscopic sphincterotomy in patients receiving antiplatelet agents—a case-control study. Aliment Pharmacol Ther 2007;25:579–84.
8. Cohen LB, Delegge MH, Aisenberg J, et al. AGA Institute review of endoscopic sedation. Gastroenterology 2007;133:675–701.
9. Vargo JJ, Bramley T, Meyer K, et al. Practice efficiency and economics: the case for rapid recovery sedation agents for colonoscopy in a screening population. J Clin Gastroenterol 2007;41:591–8.
10. Food and Drug Administration. Propofol draft final printed label. Available at: http://www.fda.gov/cder/foi/anda/2000/75392_Propofol_Prntlbl.pdf. Accessed June 1, 2008.
11. Comprehensive accreditation manual for hospitals. Oakbrook Terrace (IL): Joint Commission on Accreditation of Healthcare Organizations; 2008.

12. Aisenberg J, Cohen LB, Piorkowski JD. Propofol use under the direction of trained gastroenterologists: an analysis of the medicolegal implications. CME. Am J Gastroenterol 2007;102:707–13.
13. Trummel J. Sedation for gastrointestinal endoscopy: the changing landscape. Curr Opin Anaesthesiol 2007;20:359–64.
14. Rex DK, Overley CA, Walker J. Registered nurse-administered propofol sedation for upper endoscopy and colonoscopy: why? when? how? Rev Gastroenterol Disord 2003;3:70–80.
15. Cohen LB. Clinical trial: a dose-response study of fospropofol disodium for moderate sedation during colonoscopy. Aliment Pharmacol Ther 2008;27:597–608.
16. American Society of Anesthesiologists. ASA comments at FDA hearing on fospropofol. Available at: http://www.asahq.org/news/asanews050808.htm. Accessed June 1, 2008.
17. Aantaa R, Scheinin M. Alpha 2-adrenergic agents in anaesthesia. Acta Anaesthesiol Scand 1993;37:433–48.
18. Venn RM, Grounds RM. Comparison between dexmedetomidine and propofol for sedation in the intensive care unit: patient and clinician perceptions. Br J Anaesth 2001;87:684–90.
19. Shelly MP. Dexmedetomidine: a real innovation or more of the same? Br J Anaesth 2001;87:677–8.
20. Demiraran Y, Korkut E, Tamer A, et al. The comparison of dexmedetomidine and midazolam used for sedation of patients during upper endoscopy: a prospective, randomized study. Can J Gastroenterol 2007;21:25–9.
21. Jalowiecki P, Rudner R, Gonciarz M, et al. Sole use of dexmedetomidine has limited utility for conscious sedation during outpatient colonoscopy. Anesthesiology 2005;103:269–73.
22. Gilger MA, Spearman RS, Dietrich CL, et al. Safety and effectiveness of ketamine as a sedative agent for pediatric GI endoscopy. Gastrointest Endosc 2004;59:659–63.
23. Law AK, Ng DK, Chan KK. Use of intramuscular ketamine for endoscopy sedation in children. Pediatr Int 2003;45:180–5.
24. Kirberg A, Sagredo R, Montalva G, et al. Ketamine for pediatric endoscopic procedures and as a sedation complement for adult patients. Gastrointest Endosc 2005;61:501–2.
25. Varadarajulu S, Eloubeidi MA, Tamhane A, et al. Prospective randomized trial evaluating ketamine for advanced endoscopic procedures in difficult to sedate patients. Aliment Pharmacol Ther 2007;25:987–97.
26. Keeffe EB, O'Connor KW. 1989 A/S/G/E survey of endoscopic sedation and monitoring practices. Gastrointest Endosc 1990;36:S13.
27. Litman RS. Conscious sedation with remifentanil during painful medical procedures. J Pain Symptom Manage 2000;19:468–71.
28. Patel S, Vargo JJ, Khandwala F, et al. Deep sedation occurs frequently during elective endoscopy with meperidine and midazolam. Am J Gastroenterol 2005;100:2689–95.
29. Lopez-Gil M, Brimacombe J, Diaz-Reganon G. Anesthesia for pediatric gastroscopy: a study comparing the proseal laryngeal mask airway with nasal cannulae. Paediatr Anaesth 2006;16:1032–5.
30. Davis DE, Jones MP, Kubik CM. Topical pharyngeal anesthesia does not improve upper gastrointestinal endoscopy in conscious sedated patients. Am J Gastroenterol 1999;94:1853–6.
31. Ristikankare M, Hartikainen J, Heikkinen M, et al. Is routine sedation or topical pharyngeal anesthesia beneficial during upper endoscopy? Gastrointest Endosc 2004;60:686–94.

32. Evans LT, Saberi S, Kim HM, et al. Pharyngeal anesthesia during sedated EGDs: is "the spray" beneficial? A meta-analysis and systematic review. Gastrointest Endosc 2006;63:761–6.

33. Byrne MF, Mitchell RM, Gerke H, et al. The need for caution with topical anesthesia during endoscopic procedures, as liberal use may result in methemoglobinemia. J Clin Gastroenterol 2004;38:225–9.

34. Ayoub C, Skoury A, Abdul-Baki H, et al. Lidocaine lollipop as single-agent anesthesia in upper GI endoscopy. Gastrointest Endosc 2007;66:786–93.

35. Chen SC, Rex DK. An initial investigation of bispectral monitoring as an adjunct to nurse-administered propofol sedation for colonoscopy. Am J Gastroenterol 2004; 99:1081–6.

36. Moerman AT, Foubert LA, Herregods LL, et al. Propofol versus remifentanil for monitored anaesthesia care during colonoscopy. Eur J Anaesthesiol 2003;20:461–6.

37. Akcaboy ZN, Akcaboy EY, Albayrak D, et al. Can remifentanil be a better choice than propofol for colonoscopy during monitored anesthesia care? Acta Anaesthesiol Scand 2006;50:736–41.

38. Theodorou T, Hales P, Gillespie P, et al. Total intravenous versus inhalational anaesthesia for colonoscopy: a prospective study of clinical recovery and psychomotor function. Anaesth Intensive Care 2001;29:124–36.

39. VanNatta ME, Rex DK. Propofol alone titrated to deep sedation versus propofol in combination with opioids and/or benzodiazepines and titrated to moderate sedation for colonoscopy. Am J Gastroenterol 2006;101:2209–17.

40. Crepeau T, Poincloux L, Bonny C, et al. Significance of patient-controlled sedation during colonoscopy. Results from a prospective randomized controlled study. Gastroenterol Clin Biol 2005;29:1090–6.

41. Fisher L, Fisher A, Thomson A. Cardiopulmonary complications of ERCP in older patients. Gastrointest Endosc 2006;63:948–55.

42. Jung M, Hofmann C, Kiesslich R, et al. Improved sedation in diagnostic and therapeutic ERCP: propofol is an alternative to midazolam. Endoscopy 2000;32:233–8.

43. Fanti L, Agostoni M, Casati A, et al. Target-controlled propofol infusion during monitored anesthesia in patients undergoing ERCP. Gastrointest Endosc 2004; 60:361–6.

44. Raymondos K, Panning B, Bachem I, et al. Evaluation of endoscopic retrograde cholangiopancreatography under conscious sedation and general anesthesia. Endoscopy 2002;34:721–6.

45. Martindale SJ. Anaesthetic considerations during endoscopic retrograde cholangiopancreatography. Anaesth Intensive Care 2006;34:475–80.

46. Osborn IP, Cohen J, Soper RJ, et al. Laryngeal mask airway—a novel method of airway protection during ERCP: comparison with endotracheal intubation. Gastrointest Endosc 2002;56:122–8.

47. Fanti L, Agostoni M, Arcidiacono PG, et al. Target-controlled infusion during monitored anesthesia care in patients undergoing EUS: propofol alone versus midazolam plus propofol. A prospective double-blind randomised controlled trial. Dig Liver Dis 2007;39:81–6.

48. Agostoni M, Fanti L, Arcidiacono PG, et al. Midazolam and pethidine versus propofol and fentanyl patient controlled sedation/analgesia for upper gastrointestinal tract ultrasound endoscopy: a prospective randomized controlled trial. Dig Liver Dis 2007;39:1024–9.

49. Hammer GB, Litalien C, Wellis V, et al. Determination of the median effective concentration (EC50) of propofol during oesophagogastroduodenoscopy in children. Paediatr Anaesth 2001;11:549–53.

50. Paspatis GA, Charoniti I, Manolaraki M, et al. Synergistic sedation with oral midazolam as a premedication and intravenous propofol versus intravenous propofol alone in upper gastrointestinal endoscopies in children: a prospective, randomized study. J Pediatr Gastroenterol Nutr 2006;43:195–9.
51. Vargo JJ, Holub JL, Faigel DO, et al. Risk factors for cardiopulmonary events during propofol-mediated upper endoscopy and colonoscopy. Aliment Pharmacol Ther 2006;24:955–63.
52. Gross JB, Bachenberg KL, Benumof JL, et al. Practice guidelines for the perioperative management of patients with obstructive sleep apnea: a report by the American society of anesthesiologists task force on perioperative management of patients with obstructive sleep apnea. Anesthesiology 2006;104:1081–93.

Interventional Radiology and Anesthesia

Matthew P. Schenker, MD[a], Ramon Martin, MD[b], Paul B. Shyn, MD[c],
Richard A. Baum, MD[a],*

KEYWORDS

- Anesthesia • Interventional radiology • Quality assurance
- Sedation • Angiography

During the past the decade interventional radiology (IR) has evolved from a referral-based to a clinically based specialty. Longitudinal care now is provided to patients before, during, and after procedures. This paradigm shift has resulted in dramatic increases in the scope and volume of practice and in the complexity of patients undergoing image-guided procedures.

The need for anesthesia and procedural sedation outside the operating room (OR) continues to grow as the number of minimally invasive procedures proliferates and the complexity of cases undertaken outside the OR increases. The division of Angiography and Interventional Radiology at Brigham and Women's Hospital has witnessed a greater than fourfold increase in the number of cases requiring procedural sedation during the 5-year period ending in April 2008, with a concomitant growth in the number of cases requiring monitored anesthesia care (MAC) or general anesthesia (GA). This trend is likely to accelerate as the population ages and minimally invasive procedures continue to supplement or replace traditional open surgeries.

How are medical specialists to address this burgeoning need for procedural sedation in a safe and effective manner? Anesthesiologists are well equipped to deliver anesthesia and procedural sedation by virtue of their specialty training and broad experience in a number of settings. These settings include the OR, emergency room, ICU, pain clinic, and other procedural areas. The availability of anesthesiologists will become more limited as the demand for their expertise grows. How, then, can this

[a] Division of Angiography and Interventional Radiology, Department of Radiology, Brigham and Women's Hospital, Harvard Medical School, 75 Francis Street, Boston, MA 02115, USA
[b] Department of Anesthesiology, Perioperative and Pain Medicine, Brigham and Women's Hospital, Harvard Medical School, 75 Francis Street, Boston, MA 02115, USA
[c] Division of Abdominal Imaging and Intervention, Department of Radiology, Brigham and Women's Hospital, Harvard Medical School, 75 Francis Street, Boston, MA 02115, USA
* Corresponding author. Division of Angiography and Interventional Radiology, Department of Radiology, Brigham and Women's Hospital, Harvard Medical School, 75 Francis Street, Boston, MA 02115.
E-mail address: rbaum@partners.org (R.A. Baum).

Anesthesiology Clin 27 (2009) 87–94
doi:10.1016/j.anclin.2008.10.012
1932-2275/08/$ – see front matter © 2009 Elsevier Inc. All rights reserved.

expert resource be used effectively to maximize patient comfort and safety during diagnostic and therapeutic procedures? This article illustrates how these policies and procedures have evolved at Brigham and Women's Hospital and in the authors' division with the goals of delineating the important components of a proficient model for collaboration with the anesthesia staff and identifying future challenges facing all providers who are involved in minimally invasive procedures.

The OR model of anesthesia care is extended to procedures in the IR suite. The model of care includes

1. Adequate preprocedural assessment to determine the patient's need for anesthesia care during the procedure
2. Standardized monitoring and anesthesia equipment
3. Clearly marked and easily accessible emergency equipment (code cart, defibrillator)
4. Adequate back-up in case of emergencies or difficulties
5. Postoperative care in a postanesthesia care unit setting

With an increasing array of imaging techniques and instruments, interventional radiologists now perform procedures that once were surgical and main OR staples. In addition to regularly scheduled procedures that may require general anesthesia (ablation of venous and arteriovenous malformations, aortic endoleak repair, complex vascular stenting procedures, among others), there also are an array of emergent procedures (embolization for upper or lower gastrointestinal bleeding, hemoptysis, trauma, postpartum hemorrhage or percutaneous drainage for urosepsis and biliary sepsis, among others) that come first to the IR suite and then to the OR if necessary. These cases all require intense anesthesia care despite their minimally invasive character and non-OR venue (**Box 1**).

The difficulties inherent In IR suite procedures relate to both the technical intricacies of the procedures and the comorbidities of the patients. Interventional radiologists are relied upon to perform highly targeted, technically demanding interventions in the safest and most efficient manner for their patients. Often, interventional radiologists are asked to treat patients who cannot physically tolerate an alternative open surgery. IR treatment, however, does not mean that these "nonsurgical" candidates will not require MAC or GA for their minimally invasive procedures, a common misconception among surgical specialists who refer their patients to IR. It also does not mean that the procedure is less risky because it is not "open."

It is, therefore, increasingly common for an interventional radiologist ask the consulting anesthesiologist to assess the overall clinical picture of such "nonsurgical" candidates to devise an anesthesia care plan for the IR procedure. Assessments of a patient's body habitus and condition, underlying cardiopulmonary status, oncologic and other medical history, and various psychosocial issues are critical to both the anesthesia care of these patients and the outcome of the procedure. The determination

---

Box 1
Non–operating room locations for radiology/anesthesia

Angiography and interventional radiology

CT

MRI

Interventional neuroradiology

of the best anesthesia plan is a function of the patient's medical condition and the details of the IR procedure and, therefore, requires direct and frequent communication between the anesthesiologist and interventional radiologist.

The following discussion considers some angiographic and cross-sectional IR procedures in more detail and comments on some of the anesthesia choices and considerations. In addition, specific concerns and conflicts in the area of IR are mentioned.

ANGIOGRAPHY AND INTERVENTIONAL RADIOLOGY

The practice of angiography and IR encompasses a wide range of procedures on many different organ systems. Approximately 70% of the procedures performed are booked less than 48 hours in advance because of the relatively urgent or emergent nature of the bulk of IR procedures. Even though most of these procedures are done with a nurse providing moderate sedation and analgesia, there is a continual discussion between the anesthesia and IR staff about how best to provide for patient comfort and safety. An accurate and complete preprocedural assessment is key to having a patient comfortably tolerate a procedure (ie, hold still, breathe, and experience no pain). As a result, a member of the anesthesia team is involved in evaluating patients in far more than the 10% of IR cases that actually require MAC or GA.

Most IR procedures require that the patient lie supine. Pain from arthritis and surgical incisions, respiratory compromise from chronic obstructive pulmonary disease, pneumonia, pleural effusions, obstructive sleep apnea, and inability to cooperate because of dementia or language differences can make a seemingly straightforward procedure, such as placement of a portacath or tunneled catheter a very difficult problem in terms of the sedation plan. Some procedures, such as emergent transjugular portosystemic shunt creation, deep tissue sclerotherapy, placement of a translumbar dialysis catheter, or embolization for hemorrhage in hypotensive patients, present clear-cut choices for anesthesia care. Other procedures, such as percutaneous nephrostomies, biliary drainage, dialysis shunt maintenance, and major vessel stenting involve little discomfort after the placement of the initial access, but the patient must lie still and be able to cooperate when asked. In such situations, patient comorbidities can influence the choice of sedation and analgesia.

CROSS-SECTIONAL INTERVENTIONAL RADIOLOGY

Cross-sectional imaging modalities, including computed tomography (CT), magnetic resonance imaging (MRI), and ultrasound (US), are used to guide a variety of interventional procedures performed by interventional radiologists. The most common procedures are percutaneous biopsies, aspirations, and drainages performed in almost any body region. Many other interventional procedures, including cyst or tumor ablations, nerve blocks, and pseudoaneurysm occlusions, are performed with cross-sectional imaging guidance.

CT- and US-guided interventional procedures range from easily and quickly performed procedures requiring minimal patient cooperation and sedation to prolonged, difficult procedures necessitating patient cooperation or careful control of breathing along with significant pain control. Respiratory parameters are critical to many of these procedures because of the changes induced in target location and anatomic morphology. Respiratory motion is most problematic in procedures involving structures near the diaphragm, such as liver, adrenals, kidneys, and the lower half of the lungs. A helpful strategy in many of these procedures is to begin sedation early so that by the time initial planning scans are obtained, the patient is sedated and respirations have become shallower with reduced tidal volume. Such an approach increases the likelihood of selecting an optimal skin entry site for the percutaneous procedure.

Pain from needle biopsies varies with anatomic site and depth of needle penetration. In general, however, the level of sedation required is relatively constant throughout the needle placement and imaging phases of the procedure. With percutaneous catheter drainages, the level of pain control required tends to increase progressively from the initial needle placement through the track dilation steps and to the final catheter placement.

Percutaneous ethanol ablation is indicated for symptomatic, recurrent cysts in the liver or kidney. The initial needle placement and small-diameter catheter placement, often 6 F, usually is well tolerated, but the actual ethanol injection can produce considerable pain. Communication and coordination between the interventional radiologist and anesthesiologist therefore is needed.

Increasingly, percutaneous tumor ablation procedures are performed to manage malignant lesions throughout the body but most commonly in the liver, kidney, adrenals, lung, or bone. A variety of technologies are used, including radiofrequency ablation, cryoablation, microwave ablation, and ethanol ablation, among others. Although some ablation procedures are completed easily in less than 1 hour, completion of other cases may require up to 3 or 4 hours.

These procedures may require the precise placement of five or more needle probes into the target organ or tissue. Some radiofrequency ablation devices allow placement of a single needle probe with the subsequent deployment of an expandable array of tynes or electrodes into the target area. Other radiofrequency devices and cryoablation probes may require placement of multiple needle probes. Radiofrequency ablation accomplishes tumor destruction through tissue heating, whereas cryoablation accomplishes tumor destruction through freezing. Freezing of tissues with cryoablation tends to cause less pain than heating with radiofrequency ablation.

Regardless of the ablation technology used, reproducible levels of breath holding often are important in facilitating optimal and safe probe placements. This breath holding can be accomplished either with a degree of conscious sedation that allows good patient cooperation or with general anesthesia and same-level interruption of ventilation.

A specific problem encountered in ablation procedures of adrenal tumors or tumors adjacent to the adrenal gland is catecholamine-induced hypertensive crisis. This problem is most likely to occur when residual normal adrenal tissue is present and is less likely to occur when the adrenal is replaced completely by tumor. Radiofrequency ablation tends to stimulate catecholamine release during the application of heat to the adrenal tissue. With cryoablation, on the other hand, catecholamine release is not observed during the freeze but instead occurs during or following the thaw phase. Pharmacologic pretreatment strategies may be considered but do not necessarily prevent such hypertensive crises.

An increasingly popular CT-guided ablation procedure in the pediatric population is radiofrequency ablation of benign osteoid osteomas of bone. These painful bone lesions often are cured with percutaneous ablation, thus avoiding an open surgical procedure. Because of patient age and the significant pain associated with heating these lesions typically located adjacent to the periosteum, general anesthesia often is preferred.

MRI is not commonly used to guide IR procedures because of the many technical challenges involved in operating in an environment with a strong magnetic field. Nevertheless, the advantages of MRI, including superior soft tissue contrast, multiplanar imaging capabilities, and lack of ionizing radiation, probably will drive the increasing use of MRI for select interventional procedures. MRI guidance is favored for biopsies or ablations of target lesions not well visualized on CT or US imaging.

Positron emission tomography (PET)/CT also will be increasingly useful in guiding IR procedures when the metabolic characteristics of target lesions can be exploited for targeting purposes. The challenges of PET/CT-guided interventions include image-acquisition times of up to several minutes within a long scanner gantry and potential radiation exposure to operating personnel from high-energy radiopharmaceuticals.

As the scope and complexity of cross-sectional IR procedures continue to grow, the need for a reliable interface with anesthesiologists is clear. The use of more sophisticated sedation techniques and the formulation or supervision of an anesthetic plan of care, whether it be deep sedation or general anesthesia, is becoming increasingly important to the efficiency and success of new cross-sectional IR procedures.

ANESTHESIOLOGISTS IN INTERVENTIONAL RADIOLOGY

The unanticipated need for anesthesia support during a procedure can compromise patient safety and affect the success of the procedure. Effort therefore is focused on preprocedural patient screening. When patients who have potentially problematic comorbidities present for an elective procedure, they are sent to the preadmitting testing center for a complete assessment and are booked for their procedure with an anesthesiologist. Although this approach is time consuming, it is far preferable to a failed attempt at performing the procedure under moderate sedation alone, without an anesthesiologist present. The latter scenario creates the potential need to reschedule the case or, worse, requires an anesthesia urgent consultation or intervention while the patient is on the table in distress.

For non-elective or emergent procedures, the interventional radiologist is responsible for informing the anesthesiologist about the complexity and anticipated duration of the procedure and whether MAC or GA may be required. Anesthesiologists assigned to IR must make a crucial determination whenever they are asked to evaluate a patient for procedural sedation, namely, are there comorbid conditions that preclude the safe administration of moderate procedural sedation and analgesia by a non–anesthesia provider?

Preprocedure patient assessment in IR can be extremely time consuming and may become impossible for one individual anesthesiologist manage. Because of the increasing case load in IR and the inability to capture all relevant aspects of the patient's history, the authors use a nurse practitioner to assist with new patient evaluations in the IR suite. These evaluations include everything from routine airway evaluations to comprehensive history and physicals for more complicated patients. The nurse practitioner acts as an important intermediary between the anesthesia and IR staff. This approach allows more timely patient evaluations, emphasizing both the airway examination and, more importantly, the patient's overall clinical status. It has helped expedite the implementation of required treatments by both the interventional radiologists and the anesthesiologists.

Although preprocedure assessment is crucial, interventional radiologists also rely on the advice and direction of their anesthesia colleagues on how to perform moderate sedation in the safest possible manner and how to certify the providers who are responsible for its administration. The authors reference the revised practice guidelines published by the American Society of Anesthesiologists in 2002 for sedation and analgesia by non-anesthesiologists. This revision includes two important changes from previous editions: (1) it defines "deep sedation" as distinct from moderate or "conscious" sedation because of the greater likelihood that deep sedation could inadvertently progress to general anesthesia, and (2) it recommends that all practitioners administering sedation possess the ability to rescue patients from profound sedation or some complication thereof.[1] To fulfill these requirements, every physician and nurse in the Department of Radiology is required to maintain biennial certification in advanced cardiac life support (ACLS). They also are required to maintain biennial certification in moderate sedation and analgesia, also known as "intravenous conscious sedation." This dedicated training course emphasizes the pharmacology of agents commonly used during sedation and the antagonists used for the reversal of sedation.

IMPACT OF THE ENVIRONMENT

Nearly half the anesthesia claims reviewed by Bhanakor and colleagues[2] could have been prevented by better monitoring or improved vigilance. The most common potential mechanism for patient injury during procedural sedation is respiratory depression caused by an overdose of sedative drugs. Proper monitoring equipment is essential whenever and wherever procedural sedation is administered, because apnea events can be surprisingly difficult to identify. In one study of 39 patients undergoing MAC, 10 (26%) developed 20 seconds of apnea, but none of these events was detected by the anesthesiologists in the study who were blinded to the capnography and thoracic impedance monitoring.[3] Consequently, all patients undergoing procedures in the Department of Radiology are monitored with equipment that has audible alarms that continually assesses the essential parameters of capnography, pulse oximetry, electrocardiography, and noninvasive blood pressure. For more complex procedures or critically ill patients, invasive arterial pressure monitoring sometimes is employed. All patients have intravenous access and receive supplemental oxygen. A defibrillator is immediately available for all patients as well as a "code cart" containing the required equipment and drugs for treating a compromised airway, cardiopulmonary arrest, anaphylaxis, or drug overdose. For procedures not staffed by an anesthesiologist, the nurse administering the sedation under the supervision of the interventional radiologist records the vital signs, drug dosing, drug administration times, and the sedation level of the patient in a contemporaneous fashion on a flow sheet that becomes part of the permanent medical record. (This contemporaneous recording is the responsibility of the anesthesiologist when MAC or GA is used.) Finally, all patients are transported to a dedicated recovery room after receiving procedural sedation. The recovery room is outfitted with continuous monitoring and support equipment and is staffed with appropriately trained personnel who observe the patients until they have regained their baseline level of consciousness and are no longer at risk for the cardiopulmonary complications of sedation.

Close collaboration between anesthesia and IR has led to other workplace safety and quality improvements. For example, it was previously standard practice to maintain very cool temperatures in the IR suites because cooler temperatures were thought to be "better" for the fluoroscopy equipment. The anesthesia staff was concerned that the low ambient temperatures unnecessarily increased the risk of hypothermia, particularly in elderly and sick patients. After checking with the manufacturers, it was determined that the temperature tolerance of the equipment was 68°F, so the thermostat was reset to this level. In addition, Bair Huggers (Arizant Healthcare Inc., Eden Prairie, Minnesota) now are used for all patients to maintain body temperature during procedures.

Conversely, the anesthesia staff has learned much about radiation safety and how to reduce personal radiation exposure. All anesthesia staff are required to wear lead, and floating into and out of the procedure room without proper lead protection is forbidden. The staff also has been advised to stay as far as possible from the radiation source during fluoroscopy and to leave the room or sit behind additional lead shielding during the acquisition of digital subtraction angiography.

QUALITY ASSURANCE SYSTEM

Other authors have stressed the importance of developing safety processes and quality assurance mechanisms to track events associated with procedural sedation performed outside the OR.[4,5] Within the authors' IR division, this process starts with interdisciplinary morning rounds, in which all the patients for the day are presented via an electronic scheduling program on a large liquid crystal display monitor in the reading room. The authors use the commercial system Hi-IQ (Conexsys, Ontario, Canada), an extremely powerful and versatile system designed for the modern IR practice. Hi-IQ integrates scheduling, electronic inventory management, case-flow monitoring, coding and billing, and quality management functions. The authors use Hi-IQ to store relevant data on the patient's history, to flag patients who need an anesthesia consultation, and to track all adverse events that occur, including those associated with procedural sedation. With this large database of information, the authors can review their caseload and complications efficiently in their monthly morbidity and mortality conference, thus facilitating root-cause analysis within IR and with the Department of Anesthesia. As mentioned previously, the hospital requires biennial recertification in ACLS and procedural sedation for all IR staff. In addition, a dedicated didactic session on procedural sedation is given annually by one of the board-certified anesthesiologists.

One remaining challenge is the development of a hospital-wide system for tracking events associated with procedural sedation and integrating the data so that they can be analyzed effectively and used to determine best-practice guidelines.

SERVICE THROUGHPUT

Certainly, the liability of the interventional radiologist or any other specialist performing minimally invasive procedures is reduced when an anesthesiologist assumes the responsibility for the procedural sedation. However, the authors have noticed that overall efficiency in terms of room turnover decreases significantly in cases requiring MAC or GA. While preprocedural assessment times have been reduced with the addition of the anesthesia nurse practitioners, inefficiencies remain when trying to coordinate teams from two different departments. This disadvantage could be mitigated by an interdepartmental electronic patient-tracking program for out-of-OR anesthesia cases similar to that already employed in the main OR, but the challenge of coordinating a centralized tracking system across several different departments is daunting.

SUMMARY

IR encompasses a broad and expanding array of image-guided, minimally invasive therapies that are essential to the practice of modern medicine. The growth and diversity of these non-OR procedures presents unique challenges and opportunities to anesthesiologists and interventional radiologists alike. Collaborative action has led to better patient care and quality management. Current trends indicate that non-OR anesthesia will become a significant component of patient care throughout the hospital and will become an even larger part of the overall anesthesia practice. It therefore is incumbent upon administrators and providers to ensure that all procedure rooms are safe for patients and allow for good, consistent anesthesia practice. This article has discussed why it will become increasingly necessary to expand the scope of pre-anesthesia evaluation. As the practice of non-OR anesthesia grows, it will be equally important to develop an effective mechanism of quality assurance that tracks patient outcomes across the hospital and, ultimately, across the health system. Finally, the practice of anesthesia in the IR suite and awareness of what the practice of anesthesiology offers must be incorporated into the curriculum of an anesthesia and IR training program, because it will be a major component of all integrated practice in the future.

REFERENCES

1. Gross JB, Bailey PL, Connis RT, et al. Practice guidelines for sedation and analgesia by non-anesthesiologists. Anesthesiology 2002;96(4):1004–17.
2. Bhananker SM, Posner KL, Cheney FW, et al. Injury and liability associated with monitored anesthesia care: a closed claims analysis. Anesthesiology 2006;104(2):228–34.
3. Soto RG, Fu ES, Vila H Jr, et al. Capnography accurately detects apnea during monitored anesthesia care. Anesth Analg 2004;99(2):379–82.
4. Pino RM. The nature of anesthesia and procedural sedation outside of the operating room. Curr Opin Anaesthesiol 2007;20(4):347–51.
5. Kelly JS. Sedation by non-anesthesia personnel provokes safety concerns: anesthesiologists must balance JCAHO standards, politics, safety. Available at: http://www.apsf.org/resource_center/newsletter/2001/fall/07personnel.htm. Accessed May 25, 2008.

Radiologists and Anesthesiologists

Thomas W. Cutter, MD, MAEd

KEYWORDS

• Offsite • Anesthesia • Interventional radiology • MRI

FIRST, DO NO HARM

All patients deserve a safe and comfortable experience during a diagnostic or therapeutic radiologic procedure. Patient comfort is achieved by the gentle technique of the radiologist, with or without local anesthetic, supplemented as needed with sedative and analgesic medications. Patient safety ensues from the judicious administration of sedation–analgesia by a trained and vigilant practitioner. The definitions given by the American Society of Anesthesiologists (ASA) for the continuum of sedation–analgesia and the associated effect on physiologic function appear in **Table 1**.

The least complex procedures can be performed safely without medications or with only a local anesthetic. The next level is minimal sedation or anxiolysis, which also is low risk. If the patient requires moderate sedation, defined as sedation–analgesia that should not but could result in the loss of protective reflexes (eg, gag reflex, airway tone, ventilatory drive), additional safeguards are indicated. Among these safeguards are preprocedural preparation and evaluation of the patient, monitoring during the procedure, and postprocedural care. Guidance can be found in the ASA Practice Guidelines for Sedation and Analgesia by Non-anesthesiologists.[1] When anesthesia beyond moderate sedation is needed (ie, deep sedation or regional or general anesthesia) or when patients have significant comorbidities, a trained anesthesia provider should care for the patient.

Conducting an "offsite" anesthetic can be challenging, but the quality of care must not suffer as a result of location. Sources of risk include the patient's medical status, the procedure, the anesthetic, the equipment, and the environment. Patients should be evaluated and prepared according to the ASA Practice Advisory for Preanesthesia Evaluation.[2] Anesthetics must be provided by qualified anesthesia personnel who continually observe the patient's oxygenation, circulation, ventilation, and, when indicated, temperature. After the anesthetic, the patient must be cared for according to the ASA Practice Guidelines for Post Anesthetic Care.[3] Because support staff,

Department of Anesthesia and Critical Care, University of Chicago Medical Center, 5841 South Maryland Avenue, MC 4028, Chicago, IL 60637, USA
E-mail address: tcutter@dacc.uchicago.edu

Anesthesiology Clin 27 (2009) 95–106
doi:10.1016/j.anclin.2008.10.002   anesthesiology.theclinics.com

Table 1
Continuum of depth of sedation: definition of general anesthesia and levels of sedation–analgesia

Consideration	Minimal Sedation[a] (Anxiolysis)	Moderate Sedation–Analgesia[b] (Conscious Sedation)	Deep Sedation–Analgesia[c]	General[d] Anesthesia
Responsiveness	Normal response to verbal stimulation	Purposeful response to verbal or tactile stimulation	Purposeful response after repeated or painful stimulation	Unarousable, even with painful stimulus
Airway	Unaffected	No intervention required	Intervention may be required	Intervention often
Spontaneous ventilation	Unaffected	Adequate	May be inadequate	Frequently inadequate
Cardiovascular function	Unaffected	Usually maintained	Usually maintained	May be impaired

Because sedation is a continuum, it is not always possible to predict how an individual patient will respond. Hence, practitioners intending to produce a given level of sedation should be able to rescue patients whose level of sedation becomes deeper than initially intended. Individuals administering monitoring sedation–analgesia (conscious sedation) should be able to rescue patients who enter a state of deep sedation–analgesia, and those administering deep sedation–analgesia should be able to rescue patients who enter a state of general anesthesia.

[a] Minimal sedation (anxiolysis) is a drug-induced state during which patients respond normally to verbal commands. Although cognitive function and coordination may be impaired, ventilatory and cardiovascular functions are unaffected.

[b] Moderate sedation–analgesia (conscious sedation) is a drug-induced depression of consciousness during which patients respond purposefully to verbal commands, either alone or accompanied by light tactile stimulation. (Reflex withdrawal from a painful stimulus is not considered a purposeful response.) No interventions are required to maintain a patient's airway, and spontaneous ventilation is adequate. Cardiovascular function usually is maintained.

[c] Deep sedation–analgesia is a drug-induced depression of consciousness during which patients cannot be easily aroused but respond purposefully following repeated or painful stimulation. (Reflex withdrawal from a painful stimulus is not considered a purposeful response.) The ability to maintain ventilatory function independently may be impaired. Patients may require assistance in maintaining a patent airway, and spontaneous ventilation may be inadequate. Cardiovascular function usually is maintained.

[d] General analgesia is a drug-induced loss of consciousness during which patients are not arousable, even by painful stimulation. The ability to independently maintain ventilatory function often is impaired. Patients often required assistance in maintaining a patent airway, and positive pressure ventilation may be required because of depressed spontaneous ventilation or drug-induced depression of neuromuscular function. Cardiovascular function may be impaired.

From American Society of Anesthesiologists Task Force on Sedation and Analgesia by Non-Anesthesiologists. Practice Guidelines for Sedation and Analgesia by Non-Anesthesiologists. Anesthesiology 2002;96(4):1005; with permission.

additional equipment, and help from colleagues frequently are not available nearby, thorough preparation is essential and a system to obtain additional assistance should be in place. Although there are many methods to achieve patient comfort, the single best way to ensure patient safety is to follow the Guidelines for Nonoperating Room Anesthetizing Locations promulgated by the ASA.[4]

The environment itself can be a source of difficulty, especially when a patient is monitored from a remote location from which the anesthesia provider is excluded during the study. The patient must be observed continually, either through a window into the scanner room or a through camera trained on the patient. Vital signs also must be available immediately, again via a window, camera, or a monitor outside the scanner room.

The MRI suite may be the most hazardous location for the acministration of an anesthetic. The American College of Radiologists and the Joint Commission on the Accreditation of Health Care Organizations have established standards, guidelines, and recommendations[5–8] for the MRI suite, and the ASA is creating a specific practice advisory. Emphases include identifying patients and personnel who have ferrous implants or fragments, surgical clips, cochlear implants, pacemakers, automatic implantable cardioverter defibrillators, or implantable local anesthetic or insulin pumps and confirming safety before entering the area. Equipment labeled "MRI compatible"[9] is acceptable only if tested and labeled under the current criteria of the American Society for Testing and Materials and the Food and Drug Administration (ASTM/FDA).[8] Monitor placement and the length and routing of leads, wires, and tubing should be considered to prevent entanglement or traction as the table moves. Coiling monitor wires (pulse oximeter, EKG) have resulted in patient burns.[10] Patient temperature should be monitored during the procedure, because it may increase from the heat of radiofrequency radiation within the magnetic field,[11] or it may decrease through radiation, conduction, convection, and evaporation. Intermittent temperature monitoring may avoid the possibility of burns from the thermistor during long sessions or in critically ill patients.[12] Medical emergencies must be anticipated, and a plan must be in place. Although advanced cardiac life support may be instituted for a patient still

Table 2
Guidelines for scheduling imaging studies as awake, sedated, or under anesthesia

| | Imaging Factors | | | Patient Factors | |
Technique	Study	Duration (min)	Position	Age (yr)	Developmental Status	Coexisting Disease[a]
Awake	CT, NM	< 30	Constant	< 0.3, > 3	Normal	Minimal or none
	MRI	< 60	Constant	> 7	Normal	Minimal or none
Sedate	CT, NM	> 50	Changing	< 0.3	Normal	Minimal or none
	MRI	< 60	Changing	< 4.5	Normal	Minimal or none
Anesthesia	CT, NM	Any	Any	Any	Severe delay	Any
	MRI	< 60–90	Any	Any	Any	Any

Abbreviation: NM, nuclear medicine.
[a] Coexisting disease includes patients who have severe sleep apnea, or refractory seizure disorders, patients awaiting liver transplantation, patients who are unable to lie flat for extended periods of time, and patients who have ASA physical status 3 and 4. In addition, position may be an indication for sedation or anesthesia if it will be extremely uncomfortable for the patient an extended period of time.
From Taghon TA, Bryan YF, Kurth CD. Pediatric radiology sedation and anesthesia. Int Anesthesiol Clin 2006;44(1):72; with permission.

Table 3
Medications commonly used in radiology sedation and anesthesia

Drug	Dosage Range	Radiology-Specific Sedation Comments	Class
Propofol	150–200 µg/kg/min 2 mg/kg intravenous bolus	Potential for apnea and airway	General anesthetic
Sevoflurane	2%–3% inhaled	Potential for airway obstruction and laryngospasm	General anesthetic
Chloral Hydrate	25–100 mg/kg orally	Potential for prolonged duration of action and toxicity with impaired liver function	Hypnotic
Pentobarbital	3–8 mg/kg intravenous or orally	Potential for paradoxical reaction; can use orally in infants and small children or intravenously	Hypnotic
Midazolam	0.3–1 mg/kg orally	Adjunct; may be sufficient as single agent in severe neurologic disease	Benzodiazepine anxiolytic
Fentanyl	1–2 µg/kg	Adjunct with pentobarbital; may be useful in patients with painful condition exacerbated by position in scanner	Opioid
Morphine	0.1 mg/kg IV	Adjunct with pentobarbital or midazolam	Opioid
Meperidine	2 mg/kg IV or orally	Adjunct with pentobarbital, may be particularly useful with adolescents	Opioid
Dexmedetomidine	2–5 µg/kg/h 1 µg/kg/loading dose	Centrally acting alpha-1 agonist, with minimal respiratory depression; may be more commonly used in near future	Hypnotic

From Taghon TA, Bryan YF, Kurth CD. Pediatric radiology sedation and anesthesia. Int Anesthesiol Clin 2006;44(1):72; with permission.

in the scanner, prompt relocation outside the scanner room gives better access to the patient and is safer for the staff. If the magnet needs to be shut down quickly, the liquid cryogen boils off rapidly in a process called "quenching,"[13] and enormous amounts of helium vapor can be released, so an evacuation plan must be in place. The scanner is noisy and there have been reports of hearing loss following an MRI scan, so some form of ear protection is advisable even for unconscious patients.[14] Positioning of some patients can also be difficult, and care must be taken to avoid injury in patients who have pre-existing neurologic disease[15] or who are obese. The patient's entrance into and exit from the scanner itself warrants vigilance as well.

Interventional radiology also presents challenges for the anesthesiologist. The presence of radiographic equipment (eg, the C-arm) can make access to the airway difficult. The configuration of the table means that patient positioning, especially in the lateral or prone positions, can be problematic. The anesthesia machine and cart often compete for space with radiology equipment and supplies. Monitoring anesthetics in the CT and nuclear medicine suites poses similar problems.

ANESTHETIC TECHNIQUE

There are many ways an anesthesiologist can make a patient comfortable, but each falls into one of three categories: monitored anesthesia care (MAC), regional anesthesia (RA), and general anesthesia (GA). The choice is determined by the relative risks and benefits conferred by the patient and the procedure. MAC is the least invasive anesthetic category and is indicated when the procedure may require deep sedation.[1] The anesthesiologist provides intravenous sedation and analgesia, and the physician performing the procedure may provide additional analgesia with local anesthetic at the site. MAC is a physician service that is distinct from moderate sedation because of the

Table 4
Study durations, case turnover and incidence of side effects in children subjected to MRI under either general anesthesia (GET group) or intravenous anesthesia (MKP group)*

Variable	GET Group (n = 313)	MKP Group (n = 342)
Time to start scan (min)	9.6 (1.5)	4.2 (1.1)[a]
Duration of scan (min)	27.3 (7.9)	29.3 (11.4)
Emergence (min)	8.7 (5.5)	6.7 (4.1)
Time to discharge (min)	32.7 (10.9)	29.7 (9.7)
Whole care duration (min)	78.3 (6.3)	69.9 (7.4)[a]
Case turnover	4–5 cases/5 h	5–6 cases/5 h
Side effects		
Discontinued	0 (0)	2 (0.6)
Repeat the scan	1 (0.3)	8 (2.3)[a]
Desaturation	10 (3.2)	16 (4.7)
Laryngospasm	8 (2.6)	0 (0)[a]
Shivering	4 (1.3)	9 (0)
Total	23 (7.0)	26 (7.7)

* Data are mean (SD) or n (%).
[a] $P < .05$.
Data from Shorrab AA, Demian AD, Atallah MM. Multidrug intravenous anesthesia for children undergoing MRI: a comparison with general anesthesia. Paediatr Anaesth 2007;17(12):1191.

Table 5
Side effects in patients subjected to MRI under either general anesthesia (GET group) or intravenous anesthesia (MKP group)*

Variable	GET Group (n = 313)			MKP Group (n = 342)		
	<1 year	1–4 years	>4 years	<1 year	1–4 years	>4 years
Number	93	134	86	98	138	106
Discontinued	0 (0)	0 (0)	0 (0)	2 (2)	0 (0)	0 (0)
Repeat the scan	1 (1.1)	0 (0)	0 (0)	4 (4.1)	3 (2.1)	1 (0.9)
Desaturation	5 (5.3)	3 (2.2)	2 (2.3)	8 (8.1)	5 (3.6)	3 (2.8)
Total	6 (6.4)[a]	3 (2.2)	2 (2.3)	14 (14.2)[b]	8 (5.8)	4 (3.7)

* Data are n (%).
  [a] Significant (P < .05) compared with the older age strata within GET group.
  [b] Significant (P < .05) compared with the older age strata within MKP group and compared with the same age stratum of GET group.
  Data from Shorrab AA, Demian AD, Atallah MM. Multidrug intravenous anesthesia for children undergoing MRI: a comparison with general anesthesia. Paediatr Anaesth 2007;17(12):1191.

expectations and qualifications of the provider who must be able to use all specialized anesthesia resources to support life and to provide patient comfort and safety during a diagnostic or therapeutic procedure.[16] For RA, the anesthesiologist performs a regional nerve block. This category includes central (neuraxial) blocks (eg, spinal or epidural) and peripheral nerve blocks (eg, brachial plexus or paravertebral). GA is used when the entire patient can and should be anesthetized. For all anesthetics, patient monitoring is a critical component of the anesthesiologist's responsibilites.

Most MRI, nuclear medicine, and CT studies are associated with minimal patient discomfort. After assuring a patient's safety, the primary goal is to keep the patient still. Frequently, patient cooperation is all that is required, and little or no sedative or analgesic medication is needed. If medications are used, they should be titrated to effect, recognizing that doses that are too large may lead to confusion and disinhibition, resulting in an agitated and uncooperative patient. An anesthesiologist should be consulted if the patient may require more than moderate sedation and is at risk for the loss of protective reflexes. When a patient's medical condition is painful or if the procedure induces pain, RA[17] or GA may be chosen. If the patient is anticipated to be uncooperative during the

Table 6
Mean (± SD) values of time in minutes in the chloral hydrate, pentobarbital, and propofol groups

Times	Chloral Hydrate n = 101[a] (± SD)	Pentobarbital n = 66[a] (± SD)	Propofol n = 68 (± SD)
Sedation-ready	23.5 (13.4)	12.7 (8)	9.1[b] (6.7)
Procedure duration	48.11 (20.8)	49.3 (15.7)	58.5[b] (19.5)
Time to discharge	61.2 (31.9)	80.3 (39.2)[c]	53.9 (30.1)

[a] One patient each in the chloral hydrate and the pentobarbital groups was excluded because of sedation failure requiring transfer back to the induction room and assumption of care and further sedation with propofol by an anesthesiologist.
[b] P < .05, propofol versus chloral hydrate and propofol versus pentobarbital.
[c] P < .05, pentobarbital versus propofol and pentobarbital versus chloral hydrate.
  From Dalal PG, Murray D, Cox T, et al. Sedation and anesthesia protocols used for magnetic resonance imaging studies in infants: provider and pharmacologic considerations. Anesth Analg 2006;103(4):866; with permission.

Table 7
Adverse events after administration of the primary sedative drugs in the chloral hydrate, pentobarbital, and propofol groups

Adverse Event	Chloral Hydrate ($n = 102$)	Pentobarbital ($n = 67$)	Propofol ($n = 68$)
Cardiorespiratory events	3[a] (2.9%)	9 (13.4%)	9[c] (13.6%)
Gastrointestinal events	Emesis (2)	Hiccups (1)	0
Movement in scanner	23 (22.5%)[b]	8 (12.2%)	1 (1.4%)
Scan aborted completely	4 (3.9%)[a]	1 (1.4%)	0
Scan completed with additional/rescue sedation/Pedialyte	12 (11.7%)[a]	7 (10.4%)	1 (1.4%)
Scan completed with repositioning, bundling, or other measures.	7 (5.9%)	0	0

[a] $P < .05$.
[b] $P < .001$.
[c] Significant respiratory event in two cases referred to anesthesiologist.

From Dalal PG, Murray D, Cox T, et al. Sedation and anesthesia protocols used for magnetic resonance imaging studies in infants: provider and pharmacologic considerations. Anesth Analg 2006;103(4):866; with permission.

procedure (because of age, claustrophobia, or language barriers), then GA is indicated. **Table 2** lists the guidelines for selecting sedation and analgesia in pediatric patients based on age, developmental status, position, study duration, coexisting disease, and type of imaging study. Sedative, analgesic, and general anesthetic agents used in imaging studies include, but are not limited to, those in **Table 3**.

There is no consensus regarding the best anesthetic technique for MRI. For GA, either inhalational or intravenous anesthesia is acceptable. A scrupulous and conservative approach to airway management is indicated because of the distance and the barriers between the anesthesiologist and the patient. As with monitors, the anesthesia devices, including the airway equipment, must conform to the criteria of the ASTM/FDA. It may be best to secure the airway outside the scanner room and then transport the patient into the room. For pediatric patients, sedation with ketamine, midazolam, and propofol is adequate, safe, and comparable to that used with GA and endotracheal intubation (**Table 4**). Infants are at increased risk of adverse effects (**Table 5**) and may require a "skilled practitioner." When intravenous propofol, oral chloral hydrate, and intravenous pentobarbital were compared for anesthesia in infants,

Table 8
Frequency of adverse events occurring in five common interventional radiology procedures

Procedure Category ($n = 539$)	Respiratory Events (%)	Sedation Events (%)	Major Events (%)
Biliary procedures ($n = 183$)	8.7[a] ($P = .044$)	6.0 ($P > .05$)	2.2 ($P > .05$)
Tunneled catheters ($n = 135$)	3.0 ($P > .05$)	3.7 ($P > .05$)	1.5 ($P > .05$)
Diagnostic arteriogram ($n = 125$)	4.0 ($P > .05$)	4.0 ($P > .05$)	2.4 ($P > .05$)
Vascular interventions ($n = 51$)	2.0 ($P > .05$)	2.0 ($P > .05$)	2.0 ($P > .05$)
Other procedures ($n = 45$)	0.0 ($P > .05$)	2.2 ($P > .05$)	2.2 ($P > .05$)

[a] Statistically significant for respiratory events ($P = .044$) and any adverse event ($P = .015$) during biliary procedures.

Data from Arepally A, Oechsle D, Kirkwood S, et al. Safety conscious sedation in interventional radiology. Cardiovasc Intervent Radiol 2001;24(3):188.

Table 9
Preferred levels of sedation for all procedures

Procedure	% Awake/Alert (n Responders)	% Drowsy/Arousable (n Responders)	% Asleep/Arousable (n Responders)	% Deep Sedation (n Responders)	% General Anesthesia (n Responders)
Vascular					
Angiography	74 (163)	24 (53)	1 (2)	1 (2)	0.5 (1)
Pulmonary angiography	74 (136)	24 (45)	0.5 (1)	0.5 (1)	1 (2)
Angioplasty	62 (130)	33 (69)	3 (7)	2 (4)	0.5 (1)
Caval filter placement	67 (120)	29 (53)	3 (5)	1 (1)	0.5 (1)
Embolization	36 (71)	46 (91)	9 (18)	5 (10)	4 (8)
Transjugular intrahepatic portosystemic shunt	9 (11)	26 (32)	21 (26)	14 (17)	30 (37)
Thrombolysis	59 (118)	35 (70)	5 (9)	0.5 (1)	0.5 (1)
Atherectomy	58 (60)	36 (37)	5 (5)	0 (0)	1 (1)
Venous access	53 (78)	38 (56)	7 (10)	1 (1)	1 (2)
Genitourinary					
Nephrostomy	17 (26)	56 (85)	23 (35)	2 (3)	1 (2)
Nephrolithotomy	7 (5)	16 (11)	11 (8)	11 (8)	54 (38)
Stricture dilatation	11 (11)	33 (32)	39 (38)	7 (7)	9 (9)
Abscess drainage	33 (50)	52 (80)	12 (19)	2 (3)	1 (1)

Abdominal/pelvic				
Abscess drainage	36 (69)	49 (93)	13 (24)	2 (3)	1 (2)
Biliary drainage	12 (22)	38 (68)	32 (57)	11 (19)	8 (14)
Cholecystostomy	14 (15)	49 (53)	25 (27)	7 (8)	4 (4)
Thora/paracentesis	50 (54)	34 (37)	12 (13)	4 (4)	1 (1)
Tube procedure	47 (47)	37 (37)	13 (13)	3 (3)	1 (1)
Biopsy	62 (110)	32 (57)	5 (9)	1 (2)	0.5 (1)
Biliary dilatation	7 (10)	34 (49)	35 (50)	14 (20)	11 (16)
Gastro/jejunostomy	17 (16)	55 (53)	18 (17)	8 (8)	2 (2)
Stent placement	17 (31)	46 (83)	22 (39)	7 (12)	8 (15)
Chest					
Biopsy	67 (104)	29 (46)	3 (4)	0 (0)	1 (2)
Fluid drainage	61 (83)	31 (46)	6 (8)	0 (0)	2 (2)
Chest tube placement	45 (40)	42 (37)	11 (10)	1 (1)	1 (1)

Data from Haslam PJ, Yap B, Mueller PR, et al. Anesthesia practice and clinical trends in interventional radiology: a European survey. Cardiovasc Intervent Radiol 2000;23:259.

propofol produced the fastest induction and recovery (**Table 6**) and the lowest failure rate (**Table 7**), although the incidence of respiratory events was high. Total intravenous "light general anesthesia" with propofol and remifentanil and without airway instrumentation has been used effectively for children,[18] as has intravenous propofol alone.[19,20] The MRI suite may create the greatest challenges for the administration of an anesthetic, while nuclear medicine and CT present no special hazards aside from the location, the distance from the patient, and the radiation.

The choice of anesthetic technique for interventional radiology is procedure specific with wide variations. In adults, anesthesia for the endovascular treatment of cerebral aneurysms ranges from none to GA. Most prefer the latter to obtain optimal conditions for imaging, patient comfort and safety but recognize that GA may mask the clinical signs that guide the progress[21] of the procedure. To place a transjugular intrahepatic portosystemic shunt, MAC or GA is used;[22] The patient's mental status, ability to tolerate the procedure without moving, overall hemodynamic status, and ease of airway management dictate the type of anesthesia.[23] For the placement of balloon occlusion catheters in parturients at risk for major hemorrhage, both general[24] and epidural[25] anesthesia have been used. The epidural catheter should be placed before inserting the balloon catheter to avoid displacement of the balloon when the patient is positioned and to provide analgesia should the patient undergo a cesarean section. An endovascular abdominal aortic aneurysm repair normally requires a MAC anesthetic, although spinal, epidural, or GA are also used.[26] Before these major procedures are begun preparations should be made for emergency airway management, hemodynamic pressor support, and massive transfusion.

Relatively minor procedures, such as percutaneous transluminal angioplasty of the infrarenal aorta, can be performed safely with local anesthesia by the interventionalist.[27] Biliary tube placement or exchange, tunneled catheter placement, diagnostic arteriography, vascular interventions, and other catheter insertions have been performed using "conscious sedation" for the patient. Nurses trained in critical care can monitor the patient and administer low-dose midazolam and fentanyl (mean, 4.4 mg and 159 μg, respectively).[28] Adverse events are few (**Table 8**), and most are minor and without clinical impact. In summary, certain procedures require little or no supplemental medication, whereas others require general anesthesia. **Table 9** lists the variety of methods used for some procedures.

As with adults, anesthesia for interventional radiologic procedures in children depends on the patient and the procedure. Although sedation may be considered, GA should prevail when the procedure is lengthy or painful, when the child is uncooperative or seems uncomfortable,[29] or when the area of interest lies close to a critical anatomic structure.[30] If the child is completely covered with sterile drapes and radiology equipment impedes quick access to the child's airway, GA might be favored.[31] During placement for venous access, an air embolus may be avoided by using an endotracheal tube or laryngeal mask airway for GA with controlled ventilation.[32]

SUMMARY

Although the anesthesiologist's role in patient safety is emphasized, it should be noted that the radiologist serves the critical function of deciding whether to consult the anesthesiologist or perform the procedure alone. If the decision is to proceed with moderate sedation, the importance of vigilant clinical monitoring cannot be overstated.[28,31] Safety is best assured with no sedation, with anxiolysis, with moderate sedation with a trained and dedicated monitor, or with anesthesia administered by an experienced anesthesia provider. There should be no exceptions.

REFERENCES

1. Practice guidelines for sedation and analgesia by non-anesthesiologists. Anesthesiology 2002;96:1004–17.
2. American Society of Anesthesiologists. Practice advisory for preanesthesia evaluation. Anesthesiology 2002;96:485–96.
3. American Society of Anesthesiologists. Practice guidelines for postanesthetic care: a report by the American Society of Anesthesiologists Task Force on Postanesthetic Care. Anesthesiology 2002;96:742–52.
4. American Society of Anesthesiologists. Guidelines for nonoperating room anesthetizing locations. Approved by the American Society of Anesthesiologists House of Delegates October 19, 1994, and amended on October 15, 2003. In ASA standards, guidelines & statement October 2007. Available at: http://www2.asahq.org/publications/pc-106-3-asa-standards-guidelines-and-statements.aspx. Accessed July 30, 2008.
5. American College of Radiology. ACR practice guideline for adult sedation/analgesia. American College of Radiology. In: Practice guidelines and technical standards 2000. Reston (VA): American College of Radiology; 2000.
6. American College of Radiology. ACR practice guideline for pediatric sedation/analgesia. American College of Radiology. In: Practice guidelines and technical standards 1998. Reston (VA): American College of Radiology; 1998.
7. Joint Commission on Accreditation of Healthcare Organizations. Standards and intents for sedation and anesthesia care: comprehensive accreditation manual for hospitals. Report TX. 2-2.4.1. Chicago: JCAHO; 2001.
8. American College of Radiology. ACR guidance document for safe MR practices. AJR Am J Roentgenol 2007;188(6):1447–74.
9. Agarwal A, Singhal V, Dhiraaj S, et al. Head injury from an MRI compatible pulse oximeter. Anaesthesia 2005;60(10):1049.
10. Dempsey M, Condon B. Thermal injuries associated with MRI. Clin Radiol 2001; 56(6):457–65.
11. Bryan YF, Templeton TW, Nick TG, et al. Brain magnetic resonance imaging increases core body temperature in sedated children. Anesth Analg 2006;102:1674–9.
12. Hall SC, Stevenson GW, Suresh S. Burns associated with temperature monitoring during magnetic resonance imaging. [letter]. Anesthesiology 1992;76:152.
13. Bucsko JK. MRI facility safety: understanding the risks of powerful attraction. Radiology Today 2005;6(22):22.
14. Peden CJ, Menon DK, Hall AS, et al. Magnetic resonance for the anaesthetist. Anaesthesia 1992;47:508–17.
15. Weglinski MR, Berge KH, Davis DH. New-onset neurologic deficits after general anesthesia for MRI. Mayo Clin Proc 2002;77(1):101–3.
16. Distinguishing monitored anesthesia care (MAC) from moderate sedation/analgesia (conscious sedation). Approved by the American Society of Anesthesiologists House of Delegates October 27, 2004. In ASA standards, guidelines & statement October 2007. Available at: http://www2.asahq.org/publications/pc-106-3-asa-standards-guidelines-and-statements.aspx. Accessed July 30, 2008.
17. Gozal D, Gozal Y. Spinal anesthesia for magnetic resonance imaging examination. Anesthesiology 2003;99(3):764.
18. Tsui BC, Wagner A, Usher AG, et al. Combined propofol and remifentanil intravenous anesthesia for pediatric patients undergoing magnetic resonance imaging. Paediatr Anaesth 2005;15(5):397–401.

19. Usher AG, Kearney RA, Tsui BCH. Propofol total intravenous anesthesia for MRI in children. Paediatr Anaesth 2005;15:23–8.
20. Gutmann A, Pessenbacher K, Gschanes A, et al. Propofol anesthesia in spontaneously breathing children undergoing magnetic resonance imaging: comparison of two propofol emulsions. Paediatr Anaesth 2006;16:266–74.
21. Jones M, Leslie K, Mitchell P. Anaesthesia for endovascular treatment of cerebral aneurysms. [review]. J Clin Neurosci 2004;11(5):468–70.
22. Watkinson AF, Francis IS, Torrie P, et al. Commentary: the role of anaesthesia in interventional radiology. Br J Radiol 2002;75:105–6.
23. Connolly LA. Reply: anesthesia for transjugular intrahepatic portosystemic shunt placement. Anesthesiology 1996;85(4):946–7.
24. Sundaram R, Brown AG, Koteeswaran SK, et al. Anaesthetic implications of uterine artery embolisation in management of massive obstetric haemorrhage. Anaesthesia 2006;61(3):248–52.
25. Harnett MJP, Carabuena JMT, Lawrence CK, et al. Anesthesia for interventional radiology in parturients at risk of major hemorrhage at cesarean section delivery [comment]. Anesth Analg 2006;103(5):1329–30.
26. Kuchta KF. Endovascular abdominal aortic aneurysm repair. In J Cardiothorac Vasc Anesth 2003;7(2):205–11.
27. deVries JPPM, van Den Heuvel DAF, Vos JA, et al. Freedom from secondary interventions to treat stenotic disease after percutaneous transluminal angioplasty of infrarenal aorta: long-term results. J Vasc Surg 2004;39:427–31.
28. Arepally A, Oechsle D, Kirkwood S, et al. Safety of conscious sedation in interventional radiology. Cardiovasc Intervent Radiol 2001;24(3):185–90.
29. Hubbard AM, Fellows KE. Pediatric interventional radiology: current practice and innovations. Cardiovasc Intervent Radiol 1993;16:267–74.
30. Interventional radiology: radiology considerations. In: Bissonnette B, Dalens BJ, editors. Pediatric anesthesia: principles and practice. New York:McGraw Hill; 2002.
31. Mason KP, Koka BV. Anesthesia for pediatric radiology. Anesthesiol Clin North America 1999;17(2):479–502.
32. Yaster M. The continuing conundrum of sedation for painful and nonpainful procedures. J Pediatr 2004;145(1):10–2.

SECTION 3:
TRANSITIONAL PRIORITIES

Anesthesiology Clin 27 (2009) 107
doi:10.1016/S1932-2275(09)00027-5
1932-2275/09/$ – see front matter © 2009 Elsevier Inc. All rights reserved.

Introduction to Section 3: Transitional Priorities

Wendy L. Gross, MD, MHCM

As anesthesiologists follow the movement of cases to sites outside of the operating room, new challenges and new opportunities are bound to emerge. Some of these issues will develop simply because the environment outside of the operating room is new or different; some will arise as new technologies are encountered, and some will appear as anesthesiologists interact with medical specialists who are unfamiliar with the scope and practice of anesthesiology as a specialty.

These are all externally imposed challenges. Equally important are the internal issues anesthesiologists face as they confront their own standards and prejudices about what constitutes high quality care and safe practice.

Priorities may be challenged by the flow of cases outside of the operating room, the lack of experience medical specialists have in working with anesthesiologists and sicker patients, and the problems that arise when unprepared patients show up for complicated procedures. Economic and political pressures may intervene inappropriately, and it may be up to the anesthesiologist to stop the buck in favor of practicing quality medicine.

This section discusses important priorities that anesthesiologists must maintain as the perimeter of anesthesiology extends further from the traditional boundaries of the OR. Anesthesiology as a discipline has improved operating safety in dramatic fashion over the past 10 years; anesthesiologists must maintain their safety standards as the scope of the specialty broadens.

We begin with a discussion of the anesthesiologist as consultant: what is the mindset of a consultant as opposed to a primary caregiver, and how can anesthesiologists broaden their practices to include the need to be both consultant and caregiver? Although many medical subspecialties have resolved these questions, anesthesiologists have not. What is the best way to give advice to a medical specialist who may not understand anesthetic issues or even the vocabulary and how can one convey information in a way that is comprehensible, nonthreatening, and likely to be heeded?

We proceed to the question of pre-procedure workups and patient preparation: the out-of-operating room environment is frequently fraught with complications not found in the operating room. Procedures may involve new technologies and may be ill-defined. Anesthetic requirements may be difficult to anticipate and to accommodate in nonoperating room arenas. Procedural specialists may not anticipate the need for

Department of Anesthesia, Perioperative and Pain Medicine, Brigham and Women's Hospital, 75 Francis Street, Boston, MA 02115, USA
E-mail address: wgross@partners.org

Anesthesiology Clin 27 (2009) 109–110
doi:10.1016/j.anclin.2009.01.003   **anesthesiology.theclinics.com**
1932-2275/09/$ – see front matter

preoperative preparation; yet one must uphold the standards that have developed for intra-operative safety, which are founded upon preoperative evaluation.

The next few articles address monitoring and patient safety. Once again, transporting anesthesiology standards out-of the operating room can be difficult. Procedure suites may not be monitor-friendly in terms of space, magnetic fields, and radiograph or equipment mobility. Patient positioning may be problematic. Safety may be an afterthought, because potential dangers are unanticipated by specialists who are performing new procedures with technologically complicated equipment. What should anesthesiologists insist upon; how can anesthesiologists make their priorities consistent with the priorities of the practitioners with whom they work? Should they be the same or at least aligned? How can a common goal in terms of what is best for the patient be defined?

Finally, we discuss the anesthesiologist as intensivist and consider how the evolution of the critical care subspecialty augurs for the future as anesthesiologists outside of the operating room. The migration of anesthesiologists to the ICU occurred as the need for ventilator management skyrocketed during the polio epidemic of the mid-20th century, and anesthesiologists gradually reoriented their focus and increased their input in this arena as they defined a new role for themselves. Can anesthesiologists do the same thing with out-of-operating room anesthesiology? Can anesthesiologists become true peri-operative physicians and surgical hospitalists? The need is clearly here. The future is in anesthesiologists' hands; can it be shaped so that the specialty survives in improved form, responding to the market yet bringing our principles of optimal care and safety with us as we emerge from the operating room environs?

Consultation, Communication, and Conflict Management by Out-of-Operating Room Anesthesiologists: Strangers in a Strange Land

Jason P. Caplan, MD[a,b,*], John Querques, MD[c,d],
Lucy A. Epstein, MD[e], Theodore A. Stern, MD[c,f]

KEYWORDS

- Anesthesiology • Consultation • Communication • Conflict
- Negotiation • Psychiatry

Anesthesiology is a specialty with a comparatively rich literature examining the issues of communication and conflict. Numerous articles directed toward anesthesiologists have examined the processes of interdisciplinary information sharing and have addressed the importance of effective conflict resolution, although to date almost all of them have focused on conflicts in the operating room (OR).[1–3] Although well-developed guidelines already are in place delineating responsibilities and communication in situations such as a cardiac arrest, these rules do not apply in day-to-day consultation work, and attempts to apply them there probably will result in

[a] Creighton University School of Medicine, Omaha, NE, USA
[b] St. Joseph's Hospital and Medical Center, 222 West Thomas Road, Suite 110A, Phoenix, AZ 85013, USA
[c] Harvard Medical School, Boston, MA, USA
[d] Psychosomatic Medicine-Consultation Psychiatry Fellowship Program, Massachusetts General Hospital, 55 Fruit Street, Warren 605, Boston, MA 02114, USA
[e] Columbia University Medical Center, 622 West 168th Street, Ph 16 Center, New York, NY 10032, USA
[f] Psychiatric Consultation Service, Massachusetts General Hospital, 55 Fruit Street, Warren 605, Boston, MA 02114, USA
* Corresponding author. St. Joseph's Hospital and Medical Center, 222 West Thomas Road, Suite 110A, Phoenix, AZ 85013.
E-mail address: jason.caplan@chw.edu (J.P. Caplan).

Anesthesiology Clin 27 (2009) 111–120
doi:10.1016/j.anclin.2008.10.003
1932-2275/08/$ – see front matter © 2009 Elsevier Inc. All rights reserved.

disappointment. With anesthesiology increasingly practiced outside the OR environment, it is important that anesthesiologists begin to identify and to teach the communication skills required for practice in non-OR general hospital settings. The non-OR setting requires the anesthesiologist have both the ability to practice independently in a remote location and the ability to communicate that practice to uninitiated and often uninterested parties.

At first glance, it might seem that the specialties of anesthesiology and psychiatry have little in common. Thus, it might seem odd that the authors, four psychiatrists, have collaborated on an article intended to advise anesthesiologists on how to serve more effectively as consultants in the general hospital. The practices of anesthesiology and psychiatry have much in common, however. Both disciplines have knowledge, vocabularies, and skill sets outside the training of even the most "generalist" medical or surgical practitioner, and both have geographically distinct locations for their primary practice (the OR for the anesthesiologist, and the inpatient psychiatric unit or outpatient office for the psychiatrist). For these reasons, both specialists may be viewed as "strangers in a strange land" when they are called on to provide consultation outside the typical framework of their normal practice venue. In addition, both specialties may be asked to see patients who have provoked problems and a certain level of frustration because the team seeking consultation cannot resolve the presenting issue.

Psychiatrists, in the context of consultation, often opine on both communication and conflict resolution. Psychiatric training explicitly involves facilitating communication and the resolution of conflict, both internal and external. Psychiatry also is the only specialty that has codified a subspecialty around the practice of consultation on the care of patients who have comorbid medical conditions. Psychosomatic medicine (previously known as "consultation-liaison psychiatry") was approved for subspecialty status by the American Board of Medical Specialties in the spring of 2003.[4] Before it attained subspecialty status, however, psychiatrists had pursued advanced training in consultation psychiatry, and the field of psychiatry had long recognized certain psychiatrists as having expertise in consulting on general medical and surgical patients and to consultees on medical and surgical services.[5]

This article reviews the literature regarding practice as a consultant and the navigation of conflict and considers how anesthesiologists might apply these findings.

THE EFFECTIVE CONSULTANT

Regardless of the specialties involved, consultation involves a request from one physician (the consultee), who seeks expert clinical opinions, interventions, and treatment recommendations, to another (the consultant), who provides the requested services. Despite the apparent simplicity of this relationship, multiple factors have contributed to increasing complexity and confusion regarding the role and responsibilities of a consultant. Frequent precipitants of non-clinically motivated consultations include the fear of litigation (ie, the consultee is seeking someone to share responsibility for a difficult decision), institutional and educational policies that have had an impact on the continuity of care (ie, a consultation is generated by the primary care team because no member of the team is aware of the whole picture), and concerns about workload (ie, the consultee believes that he or she does not have time to perform the function requested of the consultant).

The authors believe that much of the frustration that some clinicians associate with consultation work can be alleviated by adherence to the steps in the consultative process listed in **Box 1**.[6,7] Specific comments regarding each element are offered.

Box 1
Approach to consultation in the general hospital

The consultant should

- Speak directly with the referring clinician.
- Review the current and relevant past records.
- Review the patient's medications.
- Gather data from family, friends, and outpatient providers.
- Interview and examine the patient.
- Write a note.
- Speak directly with the referring clinician again.
- Provide follow-up.

The Consultant Should Speak Directly with the Referring Clinician

This step seems rather obvious, but its importance cannot be overstated. Often, the official, stated reason for the consultation tells only part of the story; the real reason for the consultation and the entirety of the situation become clear only in a one-on-one dialogue with the referring clinician. Often, the referring physician does not have the expertise or knowledge to know exactly what to ask. For example, "please assist with pain management" may simply be a calling card that introduces a broader set of more complicated issues (eg, involving substance abuse, psychiatric pathology, and psychosocial chaos that the consultee would like the consultant to ameliorate).

If the true reason for the consultation is not ascertained early in the process, the consultation will not be beneficial, both the consultee and the consultant will be frustrated, and the patient will not be helped. In this era of team-based patient care and regulated duty hours, the person who actually requests the consultation may not be the person with whom the consultant talks, making it difficult to get an informed answer about why the consultation was requested. In some cases the consultant might not have the opportunity to speak to a consulting physician, communicating instead with a physician-extender: a physician's assistant, an advanced practice registered nurse, or a nurse practitioner. Once the reason for the consultation is clarified, if the consultant feels that he or she is unable to perform the requested function, or more information is needed, the consultant should discuss these limitations with the consultee, perhaps pointing the consultee towards a more appropriate course.

This response can generate no small measure of displeasure and (on occasion) outright anger on the part of the consultee, but the consultant should not feel responsible for assuaging the anxiety of a colleague. As Querques and Stern[6] have noted, "neither an ever-widening social circle nor victory in popularity contests is the [consultant's] raison d'être; competent doctoring is."

The Consultant Should Review the Current and Relevant Past Records

Even a lengthy discussion with the referring team and other personnel (eg, nurses, case managers, and social workers) does not supplant a diligent review of the written (including electronic) medical record. Especially during a protracted hospitalization, clinicians tend to organize and to summarize data in a way that may omit, or at least obscure, relevant information. They may forget to document critical clinical history and data. For example, amid the hustle and bustle that follows a traumatic accident, the primary team may forget that a patient had taken opiates for chronic pain. A thorough reading of the chart probably would uncover these lost data.

The Consultant Should Review the Patient's Medications

The consultant should make lists of the patient's current medications and those that the patient was taking before the hospitalization. It is important to ensure that medications have not been mistakenly stopped, with particular attention paid to medications (eg, opioids, benzodiazepines, and barbiturates) that induce tolerance and are associated with withdrawal syndromes. Inadvertent omissions of critical agents are common during a prolonged admission with multiple transfers between different units. When reviewing pharmacologic regimens, one should look at the medication administration record (for standing, one-time, and as-needed medicines), noting which ones the patient actually received, rather than just the medications on the physicians' written and electronic orders, because, for various reasons, the patient does not always get the prescribed medications.

The Consultant Should Gather Data from Family, Friends, and Outpatient Providers

The current caretakers, medical records, and the patient may not tell the whole story. Collateral information from others can be quite helpful in fleshing out a skeletal history, especially in outpatient settings where written information may be scant. It is important to maintain a measure of healthy skepticism, because (as troubling as it may be to acknowledge) people often distort the truth and lie.[6] For example, a drug-addled family member may exaggerate a patient's complaint of pain in the hopes that the physician will prescribe an opiate, which can then be diverted for his or her own use. No single recounting of events should be taken as definitive; each one, rather, is one aspect of a variegated history that will become clear only when all facets are assembled and appreciated as a whole.

The Consultant Should Interview and Examine the Patient

Even before the interview is conducted, the consultant has quite obtained a bit of information about the patient, but it is all secondary-source information that is gathered by others. Eliciting the history directly by the consultant expert is key, because other examiners may have missed, overlooked, or dismissed crucial data. The same principle holds true for the examination. A directed examination by a specialist consultant will be much more specific and differently focused than a general examination performed by either a generalist or another specialist. Put simply, "look for yourself."[7]

The Consultant Should Write a Note

The note should be succinct and jargon free. There is no need to rehash information that is already documented. One should write a pithy summary of what has gone on, enough to convey that the history and hospital course have been digested and understood and that the consultant's diagnosis and management suggestions account for them. The clearest and most cogent part of the note should be the impression and recommendations.[8] The impression is what the consultant thinks is going on, not just another summary of the patient's history or a recapitulation of the reason for the consultation as articulated by the person requesting it. The consultant may uncover something not evident to the consultee. Advice about management should be orderly, with ideas about further work-up (eg, imaging, nerve conduction studies, and electromyography) preceding proposals for treatment. One first should comment on the medications the patient is already taking (and suggest an increase, a decrease, or a discontinuation) and then opine on what medicines should be added to the regimen.

Suggestions should be written boldly and definitively and just as they would appear in an order (eg, "start oxycodone 5 mg orally every 6 hours"). Unless the consultant means to communicate indecision or uncertainty, the phrases "consider," "would consider," or "would start" should be avoided. These constructs drain the strength out of recommendations, and thus the recommendations are less likely to be implemented. Most often, the team already has considered these steps; what they want to hear from the expert is whether or not to implement them.

The Consultant Should Speak Directly with the Referring Clinician Again

The consultant should conclude the consultative process as it began, by communicating his or her thoughts briefly to the referral source. This step is most critical when diagnostic and therapeutic ideas are time sensitive. The consultant may not end up talking to the same person he or she initially contacted and even may have to explain why he or she is involved. Appreciating this possibility ahead of time can limit frustration.

The Consultant Should Provide Follow-up

The consultant should see the patient as often as the clinical condition warrants. This frequency can vary, but following up on one's recommendations as needed illustrates an ongoing commitment to the patient and to the consultee. If a procedure needs to be postponed pending further work-up, the consultant should suggest the course of treatment and possible timetable. To be effective, the consultant also must heed some "don'ts" (**Box 2**).

The Consultant Should not Abrogate Expertise

For the consultant to be effective, he or she must take the position that he or she is an expert and that, because of this expertise, he or she has been called in to help another physician take care of a patient.[9] Ideally, but not always, the consultee takes this position as well. The consultant does not get a sense of what the consultee wants him or her to say and then say it. The consultant is not there to "rubber stamp" an approach the consultee wants to take (or has already taken) if the consultant expert does not agree with it. The consultant cannot allow himself or herself to be badgered or cajoled into changing his or her opinion. Anesthesiologists, for example, may find it necessary to insist on practice standards that interventionalists may not understand or agree with. This insistence is part of the anesthesiologist's expert status and should not be compromised.

The Consultant Should not be Afraid to Speak Frankly

The physician's job actually is quite straightforward: "to diagnose and to treat" (personal communication, Edwin H. Cassem, MD, Boston, Massachusetts, August

---

Box 2
Some "don'ts" for consultants

- The consultant must not abrogate his or her status as consultant-expert
- The consultant must not be afraid to speak frankly.
- The consultant must not tie his or her self-esteem to the adoption of his or her recommendations.
- The consultant must not write conditional recommendations (ie, suggestions that take the form of "If this happens, then do that").
- The consultant must not be afraid to sign off of a case.
- The consultant must not forget that as a consultant her or she often is an unbidden visitor.

1999)—nothing more, nothing less. The patient has a certain disease or does not and needs certain treatments or does not. The consultant's job is to say so—whether others like it or not. In that sense, physicians are similar to baseball umpires calling balls and strikes: it isn't anything until the physician says what it is (personal communication, George B. Murray, MD, Boston, Massachusetts, September 1999). This job sometimes includes saying there is nothing wrong with the patient and that the patient does not require any medication or other treatment.[9] Diagnosing nothing may be the most important diagnosis of all.

The Consultant Should not Tie his or her Self-Esteem to the Adoption of his or her Recommendations

The team does not have to follow the consultant's recommendations. The consultees are free to adopt the recommendations or not, even if they do so in error. If the consultant's self-worth or self-esteem hinges on the consultee's following the consultant's advice, the consultant will be disappointed, unnerved, and ultimately demoralized. All a consultant can do is offer his or her best opinion about diagnosis and about treatment; unless the consultant has the authority to write orders, the consultant cannot control whether or not his or her opinions are operationalized.

The Consultant Should not Write Conditional Recommendations

First, a diligent consultant follows patients actively, and conditional recommendations are unnecessary, because when the circumstance occurs, the consultant is there. Second, the consultant cannot predict all aspects of a future event. Circumstances that were unforeseen when the consultant left a conditional recommendation may make that recommendation dangerous or ill advised. The authors disagree with Goldman and colleagues[7] who advise the provision of "contingency plans."

The Consultant Should not be Afraid to Sign-Off of a Case

Just as the consultee is not obligated to heed the consultant's recommendations (although he or she is well advised to do so), the consultant is not obligated to remain on a case and may appropriately sign-off of a case when his or her opinion and/or his or her suggestions are consistently ignored with no rationale.[9]

The Consultant Should not Forget that he or she often is an Unbidden Visitor

The patient does not necessarily come into the hospital because he or she wanted or needed to see an anesthesiologist. The patient may have come for treatment of an infection or a stroke. Now, and probably without forewarning, a physician the patient did not ask to see and does not even know is coming to see him or her and is asking a lot of questions. Even when the patient is more welcoming, it is wise to remember that, by definition, seeing the consultant is not the primary reason the patient is in the hospital. Even when the patient is admitted for a complaint associated with the consultant's specialty, the patient is not necessarily expecting to see the consultant unless the consultant is the care provider admitting the patient. The patient is expecting to see his or her doctor.

CONFLICTS IN THE MEDICAL SETTING

Physicians who work in hospitals often encounter conflict. Although conflict can involve patients and families, interstaff conflicts (eg, between consulting services or between a consulting service and members of a primary team) are among the most challenging. Unfortunately, in these situations resolution of either the underlying or overt conflict is rarely achieved. Differences in the training, culture, and philosophy of the medical specialties often create the seeds of conflict, particularly when professionals practice at the interface of two disciplines.[10–12] Collaboration, which involves the resolution of conflict, requires the creative utilization of each side's expertise, with the aim of "dismantling organizational silos"[13] rather than superficial team-building exercises aimed at the minimization of differences. True collaboration may be uncomfortable but ultimately effective, especially when conducted with civility and professionalism.

The process of resolving conflict between specialties has been described infrequently in the medical literature. In contrast, the business world actively has embraced conflict as an inevitable but potentially constructive process. Weiss and Hughes[13] (in the *Harvard Business Review*) concluded that conflict should be neither minimized nor avoided; they note that an organization can optimize collaboration only by identifying and embracing conflict. Conflict serves as an effective marker for areas where collaboration is most likely to produce the largest net benefit, because it occurs almost exclusively at the (usually unexplored and underutilized) boundary areas between different disciplines. A review of the medical literature (based on a search of PubMed databases and Medline) revealed few articles on staff conflict, and most references addressing conflict in the general hospital were limited to "dealing with the disruptive physician."[14–17]

Although psychiatrists have recognized the importance of identifying conflict in the medical setting, few concrete solutions for resolution have been proposed. In his study of interprofessional differences in the medical setting, Skjorshammer[18] identified three principal responses to conflict: avoidance, forcing, and negotiation. Of these, avoidance probably is the most common. Physicians may avoid conflict to the point of denying its existence, even when ancillary staff already have identified it clearly. Several factors contribute to the high prevalence of avoidance. These factors include personality traits that may allow success in certain areas of medical training and practice (eg, compulsiveness, perfectionism, and rigidity) and factors common to the larger system of care.[19] For example, the hierarchical nature of medical training may inhibit junior members of the team from disagreeing openly with their superiors, and they, in turn, may not learn the skills necessary to collaborate in areas of conflict. Trainees or junior staff may shy away from conflict to avoid being identified as "a problem," a designation that could affect their careers negatively. Treatment teams may attempt to ignore conflict in an effort to present a unified front to patients. As noted by Skjorshammer,[18] "when dealing with patients, they [professionals] leave behind whatever disagreements they may have." Finally, medical teams often have a vested interest in maintaining their perspective as part of their specialty's identity; to engage in open conflict may mean reformulating strongly held beliefs.

In contrast, forcing conflict is the process by which a more powerful entity forces its own agenda onto a conflicted situation without regard to the feelings of the less powerful entity. In the hospital setting, departments with perceived higher status (often those that generate substantial income for the hospital) can "afford" to ignore conflicts with other services.[18] Although this approach may accomplish the goals of the more powerful party, it generates ill will on the part of the less powerful party, who may be less likely to engage productively in the future. Forcing is, in many ways, an aggressive form of avoidance, because the process rarely includes any public recognition that a conflict exists.

The last strategy, negotiation, is the least utilized and least practiced by medical personnel. Negotiation is challenging because it requires overt acknowledgment of the conflict as well as certain skills that allow balanced and fair engagement with the other party.

Caplan and colleagues[20] have proposed a general outline for the effective negotiation of conflict in the medical setting summarized in **Box 3**. Again, specific comments on each element are provided.

Optimizing the Setting

Conflict is best addressed in person (so nuances of communication can be appreciated), rather than over the telephone, by e-mail, or via "chart-wars."[7] Less direct methods of communication provide ample opportunity for avoidance, rather than negotiation, of conflict. All parties involved should be present for the discussion so that they all can feel that they were able to voice their concerns and to avoid scapegoating of any absentees.

Identifying Points of Agreement

Parties in conflict, such as members of different subspecialty teams, first should identify areas of commonality. Doing so can help to diffuse polarities of the discussion and can clarify areas of divergence. Moreover, a reminder that each party is working toward the same ultimate goal (competent and effective patient care) can encourage a more collaborative spirit.

Clarifying Definitions

Because of differences in culture, history, and training, physicians from different specialties may use different terms to describe the same phenomenon. As noted by M.-Marsel Mesulam[21] in his text, *Principles of Behavioral and Cognitive Neurology*, "[O]ne part of the brain can have more than one descriptive name, and cytoarchitectonic (striate cortex), functional (primary visual cortex), topographic (calcarine cortex), and eponymic (Brodmann's area [BA] 17) terms can be used interchangeably to designate the same area."

Alternatively, a commonly used term might be taken to refer to broadly different concepts (eg, "decortication" may mean very different things to a neurologist and a cardiothoracic surgeon). Clarification of definitions and a jargon-free discussion can avoid conflict that may be based solely on linguistic issues.[10–12]

Disagreeing Respectfully

The most fruitful collaborations have at their roots the negotiation of conflict, which inevitably includes disagreement. Successful negotiation requires that disagreement be handled respectfully. Aspects of respectful disagreement include a full discussion of all aspects of a case, presentation of arguments in a logical and measured way,

---

Box 3
Conflict resolution in the medical setting

To negotiate conflict resolution in the medical setting, one should

- Optimize the setting
- Identify points of agreement
- Clarify definitions
- Disagree respectfully
- Maintain self-awareness
- Address issues of territory

and (perhaps most importantly) listening fully to the other person's point of view. Use of sarcasm and condescension rarely promotes respectful sharing of views and may represent an aggressive form of avoidance (ie, it may be easier to engage in a superficial bout of name calling than actually to address the pertinent issues).[22]

Maintaining Self-Awareness

Autognosis, a term that describes a reflective state both of self-awareness and of how one's emotional state might impact others, is essential to help both parties understand their reactions to conflict.[23] If, for example, one participant in a negotiation acts in a manner likely to anger his opponent, the other party might use autognosis to identify his or her reaction to the insult and not allow it to get in the way of effective collaboration. It is important that each party have a way of discharging these reactions in a safe place (perhaps a debriefing with their own team) so they can be understood and handled effectively.

Addressing Issues of Territory

It is important to address issues around territory explicitly. As mentioned earlier, conflict often occurs at an unclear boundary between disciplines, and it may be focused on where the boundary itself should be drawn. It would be unusual for a psychiatrist and an anesthesiologist to find themselves in conflict over the choice of a neuroleptic for the treatment of schizophrenia or over the choice of an inhaled anesthetic for a surgical procedure; each of these areas is contained entirely within the scope of one specialty or the other. Alternatively, the prescription of an opiate to a hospitalized patient who has a history of heroin dependence is a circumstance much more likely to generate friction between the two disciplines, because it involves aspects of each practice. Candid discussion of issues of territory, both wanted (eg, "This is my expertise, so it should be my decision") and unwanted (eg, "I don't feel comfortable taking responsibility for that") allows meaningful investigation of the issues in play and an increased likelihood of a resolution that is palatable to all involved.

SUMMARY

Feelings of frustration are central to many physicians' dislike of consultation work. Especially for an action-centered specialty such as anesthesiology, the "one back" position of the consultant, and the associated diminished sense of immediate control, can generate a tremendous sense of discomfort. When care of a patient goes awry because of ignored or inadequately followed recommendations, the consultant can be left feeling frustrated, angry, regretful, and helpless. The authors believe that the steps outlined in this article can minimize these unpleasant sequelae of unsatisfactory consultations by eradicating their most common causes: miscommunication, inappropriate expectations, and overarching (and perhaps misplaced) feelings of responsibility.

Despite all best efforts, conflict is virtually inevitable in medical settings, especially when multiple specialties (each with its own area of expertise and its own tradition, culture, language, and philosophy) are involved. Learning to manage conflict effectively can help physicians understand and embrace it with the intent of generating fruitful collaboration. Whenever possible, successful negotiation of conflict can improve multidisciplinary communication, assist in clinical management, and lead to improved clinical care.

REFERENCES

1. Lingard L, Reznick R, Espin S, et al. Team communications in the operating room: talk patterns, sites of tension, and implications for novices. Acad Med 2002;77(3):232–7.

2. Lingard L, Regehr G, Orser B, et al. Evaluation of a preoperative checklist and team briefing among surgeons, nurses, and anesthesiologists to reduce failures in communication. Arch Surg 2008;143(1):12–7.
3. Booij LH. Conflicts in the operating theatre. JAMA 2007;20(2):152–6.
4. Gitlin DF, Levenson JL, Lyketsos CG. Psychosomatic medicine: a new psychiatric subspecialty. Acad Psychiatry 2004;28(1):4–11.
5. Cassem EH. The consultation service. In: Hackett TP, Weisman AD, Kucharski A, editors. Psychiatry in a general hospital: the first fifty years. Littleton (MA): PSG Publishing Company; 1987. p. 33–9.
6. Querques J, Stern TA. Approach to consultation psychiatry: assessment strategies. In: Stern TA, Fricchione GL, Cassem EH, et al, editors. Massachusetts General Hospital handbook of general hospital psychiatry. 5th edition. Philadelphia: Mosby; 2004. p. 9–19.
7. Goldman L, Lee T, Rudd P. Ten commandments for effective consultations. Arch Intern Med 1983;143(9):1753–5.
8. Garrick TR, Stotland NL. How to write a psychiatric consultation. Am J Psychiatry 1982;139(7):849–55.
9. Kontos N, Freudenreich O, Querques J, et al. The consultation psychiatrist as effective physician. Gen Hosp Psychiatry 2003;25(1):20–3.
10. Martin JB. The integration of neurology, psychiatry and neuroscience in the 21st century. Am J Psychiatry 2002;159(5):695–704.
11. Stewart RS, Stewart M. Psychiatric interface with neurology: conflicts and cooperation. Gen Hosp Psychiatry 1982;4(3):225–8.
12. Tucker GJ, Neppe VM. Neurology and psychiatry. Gen Hosp Psychiatry 1988; 10(1):24–33.
13. Weiss J, Hughes J. Want collaboration? Accept—and actively manage—conflict. Harv Bus Rev 2005;83(3):92–101.
14. Andrew LB. Conflict management, prevention, and resolution in medical settings. Physician Exec 1999;25(4):38–42.
15. Sotile WM, Sotile MO. How to shape positive relationships in medical practices and hospitals. Physician Exec 1999;25(4):57–61.
16. Sotile WM, Sotile MO. Part 2, conflict management. How to shape positive relationships in medical practices and hospitals. Physician Exec 1999;25(5):51–5.
17. Ramsay MA. Conflict in the health care workplace. Proc (Bayl Univ Med Cent) 2001;14(2):138–9.
18. Skjorshammer M. Co-operation and conflict in a hospital: interprofessional differences in perception and management of conflicts. J Interprof Care 2001;15(1):7–18.
19. Gabbard GO. The role of compulsiveness in the normal physician. JAMA 1985; 254(20):2926–9.
20. Caplan JP, Epstein LA, Stern TA. Consultants' conflicts: a case discussion of differences and their resolution. Psychosomatics 2008;49(1):8–13.
21. Mesulam MM. Behavioral neuroanatomy. In: Mesulam MM, editor. Principles of behavioral and cognitive neurology. 2nd edition. New York: Oxford University Press; 2000. p. 1–120.
22. Jacobson SR. A study of interprofessional collaboration. Nurs Outlook 1974; 22(12):751–5.
23. Messner E, Groves JE, Schwartz JH. Autognosis: how psychiatrists analyze themselves. Chicago: Year Book Medical Publishers, Inc.; 1989. p. xix.

Out-of-Operating Room Procedures: Preprocedure Assessment

Angela M. Bader, MD, MPH*, Margaret M. Pothier, CRNA, BS

KEYWORDS

- Out-of-operating room procedures • Preprocedure assessment

Performing an anesthetic in a procedure suite instead of in the operating room can be extremely challenging for the anesthetist. Not only are the procedures performed outside of the operating room becoming increasingly more complex but also patient acuity is increasing. In some cases, the out-of–operating room procedure may be selected as a less risky alternative to an operating room procedure in an extremely high-risk patient. For example, vascular stenting procedures undertaken in interventional or neuroradiology may be preferred to open procedures in the operating room.

Effective preprocedure evaluation and preparation are critical to achieve optimal clinical outcomes and maximal operational efficiency in these areas. There are three major areas of preprocedure preparation that must be considered by the anesthetist working in these locations:

A thorough understanding of the techniques and goals of the procedure
Preparation and familiarity with the arrangement of the anesthetizing location
Appropriate screening of the patient to determine need for anesthesia presence, appropriate scheduling of providers, and medical optimization of the patient to the extent that this is possible

Many procedures performed outside of the operating room involve new technology and techniques. In some cases the procedure represents the only alternative for a highly compromised patient. It is not unusual for medical specialists to begin a procedure with an incomplete sense of what they may encounter. Clear communication between proceduralist and anesthetist is critical. If it is difficult for proceduralists to anticipate the course of a procedure, it is extremely difficult if not impossible for them to communicate next steps to an anesthetist.

Department of Anesthesiology, Perioperative and Pain Medicine, Brigham and Women's Hospital, 75 Francis Street, CWN L1, Boston, MA 02115, USA
* Corresponding author.
E-mail address: abader@partners.org (A.M. Bader).

Anesthesiology Clin 27 (2009) 121–126
doi:10.1016/j.anclin.2008.10.001 **anesthesiology.theclinics.com**

Familiarity with the physical arrangement, personnel, and operational issues of the procedural suite is essential. These suites are frequently located in sites remote from the main operating rooms. The usual resources that anesthesiologists count on may not be readily available. Many non–operating room locations were constructed without consideration of anesthesia needs because the expectation was that procedures would be performed with local anesthesia or sedation only.

The use of fluoroscopy, radiation, or nuclear MRI makes familiarity with radiation safety principles essential. Because of the need for radiology equipment and radiation, proximity to the patient may be suboptimal; these details need to be addressed when planning the anesthetic also.

The effects of the use of radiocontrast media on the patient should also be considered. Caution should be exercised when using non-ionic contrast media in patients who have pre-existing conditions, such as diabetes or compromised renal function, because nephrotoxicity can result.[1]

In addition, specific and perhaps unusual patient positioning may be required for some out-of–operating room procedures. The anesthetist needs to be familiar with these specific positioning requirements because they may result in changes in the anesthetic plan. For example, patients may be unable to tolerate light or moderate intravenous sedation because they cannot lie flat or maintain a fixed position for an extended period of time. General anesthesia may therefore be necessary. The length of the planned procedure and the level of expected discomfort must also be considered.

Anesthetists in the procedural suite may not have ready access to additional skilled anesthesia personnel should complications occur. Access to pharmacy, testing laboratories, and the blood bank may be limited. The location of a postprocedure recovery unit along with appropriate nursing resources should also be considered when preparing to work in these areas. A skilled postoperative nursing unit may be required for these complex patients; availability should be ascertained before the procedure begins. In some cases such a unit may not be available and planning ahead of time for postprocedure transport to a monitored area or ICU may need to be considered. These operational issues should all be part of the preprocedure planning, because care of the patient does not end when the procedure is terminated. The American Society of Anesthesiology (ASA) has provided some operational guidelines for structuring of these locations to ensure at least minimal standards for patient safety.[2]

The second major area of preprocedure preparation to be considered by the anesthetist is patient evaluation, which includes appropriate patient selection, scheduling, assessment, and optimization. The detailed financial aspects of out-of–operating room anesthesia scheduling are considered elsewhere in this issue. Adequate preprocedure patient assessment is essential to ensure efficient resource use. If cases are not appropriately scheduled to maximize use of anesthesiology resources, provision of anesthesia services to these out-of–operating room locations may be financially unfeasible. Appropriate evaluation and selection of patients who can receive intravenous conscious sedation by non-anesthesia care providers combined with efficient evaluation and scheduling of patients who need to have an anesthetist present results in improved patient care, maximum throughput, and revenue generation for the institution, the procedural department, and the anesthesiology department.[3]

Determining standards and developing systems for patient assessment for procedures done outside the OR is incumbent on the individual institution. Anesthesiology departments, with expertise in perioperative risk stratification of patients, have generally been asked by their institution's administrators to set forth and ensure compliance with standards for presedation assessment. Existing standards imposed by regulatory agencies or medical societies are generally not specific. The Joint Commission states that each hospital must develop specific protocols consistent with professional standards that address the following related to preprocedure evaluation:[4]

> The individuals providing moderate or deep sedation and anesthesia have at a minimum had competency-based education, training, and experience in evaluating patients receiving sedation and anesthesia.
> A presedation or preanesthesia assessment must be conducted and documented and informed consent must be obtained.
> The anticipated needs of the patient must be assessed to plan for the appropriate level of postprocedure care.
> Preprocedural patient education, treatments, and services must be provided according to the preprocedure plan.
> Before sedating or anesthetizing a patient, a licensed independent practitioner with appropriate clinical privileges must concur with the plan.

The concept that no patient should experience pain when under the care of a physician has translated to patients in procedural areas. Pain is considered the fifth vital sign, resulting in requests for consultation and assessment for pain management in numerous non–operating room locations, as stated by the ASA.[5] The ASA has stated that it is imperative for any patient undergoing procedural sedation to go through the institution's usual and routine preoperative assessment for evaluation. The ASA believes this is especially important because the patient may have only had minimal contact with a proceduralist who may have done little more than a short, directed history and examination and who may have missed major acute or chronic medical problems. In some cases, the patient may have been referred to the proceduralist who may never have physically evaluated the patient before the day of the procedure. The anesthetist or other clinician performing the preprocedure assessment may be the first care provider coming in contact with the patient who has reviewed a cardiac history, recent electrocardiograms, pulmonary and neurologic status, and other medical issues unrelated directly to the planned procedure. Failure to evaluate and optimize these coexisting conditions before the day of procedure may preclude the patient from undergoing this procedure safely, resulting in delays and cancellations.

In the worst case, if the procedure is attempted disregarding or being unaware of these coexisting medical issues, unnecessary complications can result. A closed claims review of anesthesia for procedures outside the operating room revealed that half of the non–operating room anesthesia claims occurred in the gastrointestinal suite and inadequate oxygenation and ventilation was the most common specific damaging event.[6] A significant proportion of these claims were related to patients receiving monitored anesthesia care, particularly in patients who were at the extremes of age. The proportion of death was increased in non–operating room claims versus operating room claims, and the non–operating room claims were more often judged as having substandard care. This finding emphasizes the seriousness of the preassessment issue and the need to identify patients at risk for cardiac, respiratory, and airway issues. Care must be provided that is appropriate for the patient's comorbidities, even if the procedure only requires administration of intravenous sedation.

Recognizing the need for appropriate screening is obvious; implementing protocols to identify and appropriately schedule patients who require the presence of an anesthesiologist can be difficult. It is often easy to agree on clinical parameters and protocols yet difficult to operationally implement these protocols across an institution, particularly when multiple disciplines are involved. The need to ensure patient safety, however, makes this imperative. Clinicians and administrators involved in development and implementation of these protocols need to have leadership and negotiation skills and the authority to make decisions. Implementation must include development of a quality monitoring system to provide feedback. Complications have been associated with extremes of age, increasing ASA physical status, and obesity.[7]

The ASA Task Force on Sedation and Analgesia by Non-Anesthesiologists has developed guidelines to assist in the development of institutional policies and procedures to help ensure safe preprocedural assessment practices.[8] The task force recommended that clinicians administering sedation should be familiar with the depth of sedation required for the particular procedure and with aspects of the patient's medical history that might alter the patient's response to sedation and analgesia. The presence of these factors may trigger involvement of an anesthetist to determine whether a non-anesthesiologist can perform the sedation or whether the patient factors warrant that an anesthetist should be present. These factors include:

Patients who have abnormalities of the major organ systems

Patients who have had previous problems with anesthesia or sedation

Patients who have a history of stridor, snoring or sleep apnea

Patients who have dysmorphic facial features, such as Pierre Robin syndrome or trisomy 21

Patients who have oral abnormalities, such as a small opening (<3 cm in an adult), edentulous, protruding incisors, loose or capped teeth, high arched palate, macroglossia, tonsillar hypertrophy, or a nonvisible uvula

Patients who have neck abnormalities, such as obesity involving the neck and facial structures, short neck, limited neck extension, decreased hyoid-mental distance (<3 cm in an adult), neck mass, cervical spine disease or trauma, tracheal deviation, or advanced rheumatoid arthritis

Patients who have jaw abnormalities, such as micrognathia, retrognathia, trismus, or significant malocclusion

Patients receiving significant amounts of pain medication chronically or who for other reasons may be tolerant to agents used during sedation and analgesia

The ASA recommends that preprocedure testing be guided by the patient's underlying conditions and the likelihood that the results will alter the management of sedation and analgesia. The ASA also recommends that patients or their legal guardians be informed of and agree to the administration of moderate and deep sedation. Risks, benefits, limitations, and alternatives should be discussed and signed informed consent obtained. The task force agreed that preprocedure fasting decreases risks during sedation. The same fasting guidelines used for operating room procedures with anesthesia can be applied.

A similar task force was convened to address preprocedure guidelines for pediatric patients receiving sedation for diagnostic and therapeutic procedures.[9] These recommendations for pediatric sedation include documentation of informed consent, provision of education and instructions to the responsible person, and documentation of preprocedure health evaluation.

The health evaluation for both pediatric and adult patients should be performed by an appropriately licensed practitioner and reviewed by the sedation team at the time of treatment for possible interval changes. This evaluation should document baseline status and specific risk factors that may warrant additional optimization before the procedure. Specific factors as noted previously may warrant the presence of an anesthetist skilled in advanced airway management, in advanced cardiovascular management, or in dosing particular types of medication not familiar to the non-anesthetist.

The health evaluation should include a careful list of allergies and current medications, including over-the-counter medications that may interfere with other agents. Particular care should be paid to diseases, physical abnormalities, and neurologic impairments that may increase the risk for airway obstruction; many of these are included in the list provided previously. Pregnancy status, relevant previous hospitalizations and surgeries, relevant family history, and a history of response to previous sedation and anesthesia should be elicited and documented. The review of systems should focus on organ system dysfunction that may alter the response to sedation or put the patient at risk for instability during the procedure. A focused physical examination with attention to the airway, heart, and lungs should be documented. An ASA physical classification should be assigned. Consultation with an anesthesia care provider may be helpful in some ASA class III and likely all ASA class IV patients.

When performing an anesthesia evaluation for cases occurring outside the operating room, it is important to remember that personnel in many of these locations may not be educated about anesthesia needs. It is therefore essential to document all special issues so that anesthesia personnel can be forewarned and plan appropriately. At the Brigham and Women's Hospital in Boston it has been our practice to communicate these issues by e-mail to the scheduling office so that they can be forwarded ahead of time to the anesthesia team assigned to the case. These issues may include conditions such as morbid obesity, difficult airway, pregnancy, and significant cardiac or pulmonary issues. The assigned team can then appropriately prepare to deal with all of these issues in an area that may be remote from the operating room.

Although there is agreement that the preprocedure evaluation must be performed, the depth and timing of this evaluation is extremely variable. In many cases the proceduralist may not have met the patient in person before the day of the planned procedure. Clerical or clinical people may do various phone screens; patients may not be triaged appropriately to the preanesthesia evaluation clinic. Inappropriate screening can result in inability to identify patients who require anesthesia consultation or presence of an anesthesiologist during the procedure. In these cases several undesirable outcomes may occur. Patients may arrive on the day of procedure only to be cancelled if the preprocedure evaluation reveals unresolved medical issues. Patients may have unnecessary pain during the procedure if they have a history of high tolerance to pain medication and a non-anesthesiologist who is limited in the total amount of drug that can be given performs the sedation. Untoward complications may occur if personnel untrained to manage complex medical comorbidities or airway abnormalities attempt to perform intravenous sedation without an anesthesiologist present. Because scheduling of anesthesia staff must be done in a way to maximize use and efficiency, most groups do not have free personnel available to provide care for elective outpatient procedures when the cases have been inappropriately scheduled without an anesthesiologist and problems are recognized when the patient presents for the procedure. For all of these reasons, it is imperative that each institution develops appropriate pathways for triage for these patients. These pathways should address patients who are seen in a clinic by the proceduralist ahead of time and patients who are referred by outside physicians and are not seen by the proceduralist until the day of the procedure. The proceduralist and the referring physicians should be provided with algorithms to identify patients who may be at higher risk for sedation and who may need consultation in the institution's preoperative clinic. These evaluations will determine whether an anesthesiologist needs to be present for the procedure and provide required documentation of anesthesia assessment when it is known that anesthesia is required. Moreover, clinic visits also provide a pathway for medical issues to be resolved, laboratory results to be reviewed, and medical optimization to occur. In selected high-risk patients, patients residing in nursing homes, or patients referred from long distance, mechanisms should be developed to send existing medical information to the preoperative clinic for review so that no issues will preclude performing the procedure on the date scheduled. In addition, this preemptive planning ensures that an anesthesiologist is scheduled and available for all appropriate cases. Excellent interdisciplinary collaboration is required for these algorithms to be developed and implemented throughout the institution.

In summary, the need to provide analgesia and anesthesia for patients having procedures outside the operating room continues to increase. The increasing complexity and scope of the procedures performed and the growing acuity of this patient population make it imperative from a quality standpoint that institutions develop and consistently implement appropriate algorithms. Pathways must be generated to identify factors that make patients higher risk. These pathways should also lead to efficient scheduling and resource use with optimal clinical and operational outcomes for all involved.

REFERENCES

1. Parfrey PS, Griffiths SM, Barrett BJ, et al. Contrast-induced renal failure. N Engl J Med 1989;320:143–9.
2. American Society of Anesthesiology. Guidelines for nonoperating room anesthetizing locations. Available at: http://www.asahq.org/publicationsAndServices/sgstoc.htm. Accessed August 2008.
3. Dexter F, Xiao Y, Dow AJ, et al. Coordination of appointments for anesthesia care outside of operating rooms using an enterprise-wide scheduling system. Anesth Analg 2007;105:1701–10.
4. Joint Commission. Refreshed Core. Available at: http://www.jointcommission.org/. Accessed August 2008.
5. Leak JA. Hospital-based anesthesia outside the operating room. American Society of Anesthesiology Newsletter 2003;67(10): Available at: http://www.asahq.org/Newletters/2003/10_03/leakIntro.html. Accessed August 2008.
6. Robbertze R, Psner KI, Domino KB. Closed claims review of anesthesia for procedures outside the operating room. Curr Opin Anaesthesiol 2006;19(4):436–42.
7. Pino RM. The nature of anesthesia and procedural sedation outside of the operating room. Curr Opin Anaesthesiol 2007;20(4):347–51.
8. Gross JB, the American Society of Anesthesiologists Task Force on Sedation and Analgesia by Non-Anesthesiologists. Practice guidelines for sedation and analgesia by non-anesthesiologists. Anesthesiology 2002;96:1004–17.
9. Cote CJ, Wilson S, The Work Group on Sedation. Guidelines for monitoring and management of pediatric patients during and after sedation for diagnostic and therapeutic procedures: an update. Pediatrics 2006;118:2587–602.

Patient Safety: Anesthesia in Remote Locations

Allan Frankel, MD

KEYWORDS

- Teamwork • Leadership • Remote locations
- Outpatient anesthesia • Anesthesia safety

The safety of anesthesia delivered in the operating room is enhanced by the standardization and reliability built into that environment, which has prescriptive and detailed protocols for almost every procedure performed. Although operating rooms allow for variation based on surgical and anesthesia preference, there is excellent overall management of the technical aspects of surgery. Experienced anesthesiologists come to rely on these operating room characteristics to support the delivery of safe care. Anesthesiologists giving anesthesia outside the operating room often find themselves in settings that lack this rigor and that therefore challenge safety.

The decreased safety of anesthesia administration outside of operating rooms can result from

Working with individuals who do not understand the nuances of anesthetic management and may not appreciate the fine line between a stable and uneventful case and a potentially dangerous or lethal one

Less efficient or effective scheduling, resulting in inefficient or hurried patient preparation

Equipment that is less well maintained than in the operating room

Greater variation in physical set-ups and anesthesia and monitoring equipment, resulting in the anesthesiologist's decreased familiarity with the environment and the equipment

Greater variability in the time needed to obtain patient records, which can cause delays in collecting adequate information about patient history and the procedures to be performed

Inadequate monitoring of stock items, which therefore may be missing or in short supply

Nursing and support personnel who do not follow rigorous preprocedure check-in processes

Working with individuals whom the anesthesiologists has not met before or does not know well

Principal Pascal Metrics Inc., 3050 K Street NW, Suite 205, Washington, DC 20007, USA
E-mail address: afrankel@pascalmetrics.com

Anesthesiology Clin 27 (2009) 127–139
doi:10.1016/j.anclin.2008.10.005
1932-2275/08/$ – see front matter © 2009 Elsevier Inc. All rights reserved.

Being at a distance from the core areas where anesthesiologists congregate, so less local support is available when problems arise, there are fewer opportunities to discuss questions or concerns, and there are fewer opportunities to collaborate if problems appear

Some of these shortcomings can be addressed by interdepartmental planning by staff in the remote location before the anesthesiologist delivers the anesthetic for the first time. Other shortcomings require the anesthesiologist's or certified registered nurse anesthetist's ongoing or daily attention when arriving to perform a procedure. This article describes the basic concepts in safety and then applies them to these two aspects of ensuring safe care in remote locations.

ANESTHESIA AS A SYSTEM

For the purposes of this explanation, one can consider anesthesia in a remote location as a complicated "system" with numerous associated characteristics. This system begins when an anesthesiologist or other anesthesia practitioner leaves the predictability of the operating room and ventures into a remote location and ends when the anesthetic has been delivered and the practitioner hands off responsibility for that patient.

Safety and Reliability

Safety is an attribute of the remote anesthesia system that often is defined clinically as the likelihood that the anesthetic can be delivered in a manner that achieves the desired goal and causes no harm to the patient.

In addition to this clinical perspective, safety can be considered from an engineering perspective that delves deeply into the components of delivering anesthesia from a remote location and considers

The reliability of achieving the desired outcome, not just once but repeatedly
Evaluating the processes leading to the desired outcome
Analyzing in detail the indivisible steps that, together, make up the process

The process has dozens and in some cases hundreds of sequential steps. The reliability of each of the steps—that is, whether each step occurs as it should—determines whether the desired outcome is achieved.

Ultimately, system safety and reliability are determined by the rate of defects in each step. When defect rates are multiplied, it becomes increasingly likely that they will lead to an undesired outcome. The result could, but not always, be clinical harm to the patient. The patient may be fine, but the process nevertheless may have significant flaws that predispose patients to a greater-than-reasonable risk of harm. Although the current patient did not suffer an adverse event, the next patient might not be so lucky.

If the anesthesiologist's clinical perspective is combined with the engineer's perspective, a reliable anesthetic performed in a remote location will see the patient safely through the procedure because all of the steps in the processes have reliably small and known defect rates.

Process Steps

To take this theoretical construct and make it real, one should consider that each step in the process (eg, when an anesthesiologist in a remote location gets the patient's chart) is an individual and indivisible action. The simple act of holding the chart in one's hands is a step in the process of evaluating the patient before administering an anesthetic.

Once the chart is in hand, a series of other steps might include checking the hematocrit box in the laboratory section of the chart, checking the consent box in the front of the chart, and perusing the blood pressure and heart rate trends in the clinical section. These actions comprise three more steps (or four, if blood pressure and heart rate are on different pages of the clinical section of the chart) that each depend on a number of previous processes (eg, the secretary or nursing assistant placing the chart in a location convenient to the anesthesiologist and checking that the correct information is in the correct place in the chart). The process steps undertaken by the secretary and the nursing assistant each have failure rates also and determine whether the information is present in the chart when it reaches the anesthesiologist.

Suffice it to say that giving an anesthetic in any location, viewed from this perspective, is made up of dozens to hundreds or thousands of steps, and every one of them has an intrinsic defect rate; some might be single steps, but many have associated processes that determine their defect rate.

To the degree that each of the steps' defect rates can be quantified, the safety of a system is measurable, and the measure is not only whether the outcome is achieved but whether the processes can be replicated. To a large extent, safety is a system property determined by the system's reliability.

ACHIEVING RELIABILITY IN SYSTEMS

Anesthesia has done a remarkably good job of making itself reliable, albeit in a health care industry that has been slow to incorporate many key features of reliable systems. The Harvard Anesthesia Practice Standards[1] generated in the 1980s and adopted across the United States is an example of the standardization of anesthesia care that has helped improve the safety of the specialty. These standards identified minimum monitoring expectations now commonly used in every anesthetic procedure and influenced the broad adoption of pulse oximetry and capnography.

Another rich source of reliability in the field of anesthesia is derived from promoting the interoperability of anesthesia practitioners. Although one anesthesiologist may begin a procedure, it is likely that any other member in a department would be capable of replacing him or her if called upon to do so. This exchange is likely in many departments in which transfers of care occur daily.

The interoperability of anesthesia practitioners is not a function solely of the anesthesiologist's somewhat brief relationships with patients as compared with other specialists but has been adopted because it allows greater flexibility and, ultimately, confers greater reliability to the departments that adopt it.

Reliability is feasible only when a group of interdependent factors are woven together effectively to produce a whole cloth. The threads are the key; their individual quality determines the quality of the final tapestry. There are five types of threads in the weave:

An environment of continuous learning
A just and fair culture
An environment of enthusiasm for teamwork
Leaders engaged in safety and reliability through the use of data
Effective flow of information

Weaving occurs only through concerted effort at multiple levels, starting with a desire to achieve reliability as the goal that takes precedence over all others. Organizations and departments that embark on the road to greater reliability find that the end result positively influences patient care and employee satisfaction and even is obvious to outside observers. To some extent this sense of reliability applies to anesthesia practitioners as they arrive in a remote location to participate in a procedure. The initial reaction, that gut feeling about the quality of relationships and the safety of the environment, should be taken seriously, because it is likely to be a fairly good indicator of the risk inherent in the environment.

An Environment of Continuous Learning

The paradigm of a learning environment is Toyota Industries.[2] The company leads the automobile industry in size and sales, and the enthusiasm of their car owners is well known. Toyota employees make suggestions for improving the work they do an average of 46 times per year and do so with the knowledge that a significant number of their suggestions will be tested and, if found worthy, adopted and spread. This process of applying the insights of the front-line workers to change and improvement applies not only to the production of their cars, it applies to the fundamental work of improvement itself. Toyota not only strives continuously to improve its car production, it strives to improve the way it makes improvements. In other words, if a change in a procedure takes 1 month today, Toyota seeks ideas so that a year from now it could perform that change in 3 weeks. If Toyota daily receives 10 useful suggestions from a department, then its goal is to receive 12 or 15 suggestions 1 year from now. Its perspective is that improvement always is feasible, and there always is waste to be removed from its processes. The fact that in a prior quarter wasted effort and materials decreased as a result of focused improvement efforts is immaterial. There is, unrelentingly, always more to be achieved.

Where is health care in this picture and how does the example of Toyota apply to anesthesiologists when they arrive in a remote location to give an anesthetic? Physicians and hospitals have, for decades, had a guild relationship in which individual physicians plied their trade within the walls of a hospital but with singularly insular perspectives. In the last 20 years a different health care industry has begun to emerge, built on hard evidence from randomized, controlled clinical trials. Groups of clinicians now provide service line delivery across the spectrum of care associated with specific diseases.

An environment of continuous learning in health care requires the presence of certain structural elements and the ability to execute ideas. The most basic of structural elements is the meeting of the clinical, unit-based leadership to consider information about unreliable events and decide on actions to remedy them. Anesthesia in sites remote from the operating room can take place safely only in clinical units whose leaders are able to orchestrate this process, and anesthesia must be an integral part of the structural elements in that unit. For example, members of a gastroenterology suite consider how to use conscious and deep sedation and, occasionally, general anesthesia. The staff of a multidisciplinary group should meet on a regular basis to examine the straightforward operational issues in the unit, from items as specific as getting drugs to the right places in each room to the flow of patients through the entire suite. Anesthesia representation in these meetings ensures that anesthetic issues are addressed appropriately.

The information collected at such meetings should be collated and evaluated so that remedies to any problems, potential problems, or concerns may be pursued. As in Toyota and other companies with reputations for high reliability, listening to the front line and acting on its concerns is a key to ensuring a safe process. Requisite are an environment or culture that makes it easy to bring problems to light and a teamwork structure that supports this process. Both these elements can be evaluated.

A Just and Fair Culture

A just and fair culture in health care is one in which individuals fully appreciate that although they are accountable for their actions, they will not be held accountable for system flaws. Their full appreciation of this distinction means they believe (and that their belief is corroborated by the actions of the organization and their peers) that a reasonable mechanism exists for evaluating untoward events, regardless of the outcome of the event. Implicit in this belief, and an extension of it, is that actions are evaluated based on what is best for the patient and not on who is supporting the actions. Hierarchy, whether formal or informal, is not material in discussions of this sort.

Thoughtful experts on both sides of the Atlantic have developed schema to address this topic. James Reason in the early 1990s described his Incident Analysis Tree.[3] In the last decade David Marx developed his "Just Culture Algorithm"[4,5] for evaluating the choices made by front-line providers, which both incorporates and expands on Reason's work. In both cases the goal is to ensure appropriate accountability and an environment in which every decision made by senior leadership and middle management is based on integrity and ethics.

In assessing levels of culpability in some serious patient injuries, there are contributing factors about which agreement is universal. Other individual actions or events may require careful analysis, teasing away bias or misconception, to arrive at a conclusion that the majority will find fair and just. These are the gray areas in the analysis, lacking the discrete black and white forms and shapes that, if always present, would make this process much more straightforward.

The advantage of promoting, nurturing, and supporting a climate perceived as fair is that it opens the doors for discussion about problems and makes it acceptable to explore opportunities for improvement, to disagree, and to find resolution through testing and the quest for continuous improvement. A culture of fairness is a fundamental to the implementation of a safe system. Although the prevailing culture probably is not foremost the issue on an anesthesiologist's mind as he or she inserts an endotracheal tube in a radiology or gastroenterology suite, a culture, fair and just or otherwise, is present every time a tube is inserted and will, in part, determine the degree to which the environment supports the safety of each insertion.

An Environment of Enthusiasm for Teamwork

Debriefing: a teamwork behavior that marries team practice and improvement
There are only a few core team behaviors. An unlikely one to start with, but ultimately one of the most important, is debriefing. This one practice alone, if conducted routinely in a unit with the appropriate structural supports as described so far, would make remote anesthesia generally safe.

Debriefing is the simple practice of convening the team immediately after finishing a procedure (or a series of procedures) to ask and answer three simple questions:

What did we do well?
What could we have done better?
Did we learn anything that we should take into account for the next procedure?

If performed well, with experience and an agreed-upon protocol, the debriefing can generate essential information in less than 2 minutes. Once the debriefing discussion has occurred, the next set of steps, those that support the debriefing act, ultimately are more important than the debriefing itself. In this phase the information is funneled to the unit so that an improvement process can be considered and its findings acted upon.

Debriefings and the supporting structure are simple concepts but often are hard to put into practice. They require engaged and knowledgeable leadership, team buy-in, and the ability to analyze information and formulate process improvement actions. Debriefings and the supporting structure make the difference between a stellar unit and a mediocre one. The process is so important that every unit or clinical department should articulate a core value to describe it and then establish norms of conduct shaped by that value. The value could be stated as simply as "endless learning" and the norm of conduct an expectation that every team member will participate in the debriefing. The expectations of leadership shine brightest here. If team members do not take on the expected norms of conduct, a series of proscribed steps must be followed that ultimately, and only if necessary, lead to the removal of that team member. This process is not one for the faint of heart to undertake, but for leaders who want to be effective, it is essential.

Determining how to make debriefings a natural part of anesthesiologists' clinical environments is not part of most clinicians' thinking. Most clinical environments where anesthesia now is practiced are not configured to undertake debriefings, but only because there is insufficient appreciation of their value, inadequate understanding about how to do them efficiently, and incomplete knowledge of what to do with the information. Productivity-centered units and departments leave little or no time for even the briefest reflection. In fact, when debriefing occurs, it is usually in the aftermath of a severe adverse event, and even these debriefings are conducted in a manner that is not likely to generate the best results.

Evaluations of severe adverse events should be conducted as soon as possible after the event. After 24 the participants' minds begin to fill in the memory's blank or gray areas, reshaping the events to meet all manner of personal predispositions, to help protect oneself or explain away the uncomfortable. Effective debriefing will occur at the most critical times only if it is practiced in the most mundane of times—in the debriefings that occur after a day's normal and successful activities. Daily, routine debriefings provide the opportunity to highlight the good work done by the team and group and always create the opportunity to learn something about how to make the work better.

Operating rooms in the United Kingdom, the United States, and Canada are experimenting with debriefing as part of team-training efforts and through collaboratives run by the Institute for Health care Improvement. Almost every site is struggling with aspects of the debriefing, beginning with the question of when to do them. Most of those who have been successful have settled, to begin with, on a debriefing process that occurs in general anesthetics between the time skin closure begins and the time just before the patient emerges. There is no ideal time for this activity to occur, but at this time all the operating room participants tend to be together, and there usually is a moment of stability and calm before the patient emerges. The debriefing discussion, if done well, can be as brief as 120 seconds. If the session is well coordinated, and if each member of the team understands its purpose, the debriefing can yield an extraordinary amount of information.

In a culture in which debriefing is fully developed and routinely practiced, members of the team might, in real time, notice aspects of the procedure that are worthy of mention and tuck them away mentally until the debriefing takes place. The result is a rapid debriefing discussion about things that went exceptionally well and should be repeated, those that were problematic and need to be fixed, and insights that might be fodder for future improvement tests. In such a setting, because the team members are used to the debriefing drill, they know who gets to speak up first (always the most junior member or the individual with the least authority), and they know how to express the issues and in what order. A team member has the assigned responsibility of collecting the information on a form, which in a well-developed scenario is readily and easily accessible, and that individual—whether the surgeon, nurse, technician, or anesthesia practitioner—knows where to deposit the form. Team members also know that the form serves a useful purpose, that the comments noted on the form are evaluated by departmental leaders, and that the comments are taken seriously. They see changes take place as a result of the comments, and they receive direct feedback when a specific comment they have made is acted upon. Of course, for that feedback to occur, the well-designed collection instrument has a place for individual's names so that leaders know where the comments originate, which procedures are being commented upon, and what time of day the comments are made. Not every form needs to have all of this information; if a provider decides to pick up a form and insert an anonymous comment, that procedure is acceptable, too. The culture is one of fairness so that providers are not hesitant about adding their names to the concerns expressed by others.

THE GOOD HEALTH CARE TEAM

What is a good health care team? A good team is a group of interdependent individuals who have the following characteristics:

They have diverse skills and share a common goal.

Their output, through synergy, is greater than the sum of the individuals within the group.

They have an appreciation of the roles played by each team member, including the leaders.

They know each other's expertise so well that that team members know where to turn to solve a problem.

They have each agreed, individually, on norms of conduct, one of which is non-negotiable mutual respect.

They address technical problems directly using the skill mix of the team, but they face complex problems that require adaptation and flexibility through collaboration and open discussion.

Individuals may express concerns without fear of retribution and know that their concerns will engender only two possible responses: either their concerns will be acted upon, or knowledge that mitigates the concern will be brought to light respectfully.

Excellent teams have team leaders who clarify, each time the team comes together, the expected norms of conduct. In addition to having agreed-upon norms of conduct, outstanding teams have the added support of organizational endorsement.

Outstanding leaders help frame norms of conduct by choosing a few values that guide the organization as a whole. Value statements become useful in this context (eg, from Ascension Health: "Health care that works, Health care that is safe, Health care that leave no one behind,"[6] and from the Mayo Clinic "Always in the patient's best interests").[7]

TEAM LEADERSHIP

Team leadership is not an innate skill; it is learned. Physicians are, by definition, the leaders of their teams, and nowhere more so than in the environments where general anesthesia is performed. Shared leadership between the anesthesia practitioner and the surgeon or specialist is essential in the operating room and in remote locations and is feasible only with some forethought, some discussion about agreed-upon norms of behavior, and with practice.

One act of good leadership is to take the team through a process called "briefing." Unlike terms such as "pause" or "time-out," briefing is not a static, one-time event. Briefing is an ongoing process that ensures that that all team members have a similar mental model of the team's expected actions and assumes that, as the plan changes or requires changing, team members will be informed and engaged in making informed decisions.

Briefings in operating rooms are multistep affairs, ideally beginning with a coming together of the surgical team with the patient in the preoperative area and a discussion that engages the patient and team members in delineating the plan for that procedure. The briefing process might continue after the patient is sedated or asleep in the operating room, at which point a further briefing might ensue about any issues that team members might consider unsettling. These issues might include, for example, concerns about equipment logistics or a team member's personal comments about what he or she feels are his or her limitations that day, stated as a request for more support from other team members. In the United States a third part of the briefing process occurs just before incision and is called the "time-out." This step is a regulatory requirement to ensure correct laterality of the procedure and identification of the patient and procedure.

A good initial briefing process has four components in which leaders

Ensure that all team members know the plan for the procedure

Assure team members they are operating in an environment of psychologic safety, where they may be completely comfortable speaking up about their concerns

Remind team members of agreed-upon norms of conduct, such as specific forms of communication that increase the likelihood of accurate transmission and reception of information

Expect excellence and excellent performance, reminding team members of their responsibility to do their best and remain, throughout, engaged in the performance of the team activity and centered on the game plan and team goals

A briefing will be only as good as the team leader who runs the briefing. In general physicians are not trained to run briefings, nor have they trained health care front-line providers to participate in briefings. The result in operating rooms is likely to be evident to every practitioner reading this article: the classic experience of anesthesiologists and surgeons schooled to believe in individual autonomy and the presumption of excellence, which leads to the scenario of the anesthesiologist walking into an empty room in a remote location and setting up his or her equipment. Then, at the appointed time, or often delayed and later, a nurse enters with a patient. At that time a dance begins between the nurse, anesthesia practitioner, and patient to gather the appropriate data and position the patient for anesthesia. Some time after that the surgeon or specialist arrives and may or may not acknowledge the presence of other team members, his or her behavior scripted on the assumption that everyone in the room is an expert in his or her field and that if everyone does what he or she is supposed to do, the job will get done safely. Discussion is limited; if there is any, it involves issues unrelated to the procedure, once again because of the assumption that everyone knows his or her job so that discussion about the work is redundant, might be an affront to the skills of the practitioners, or a waste of time. Nothing could be further from the truth.

Briefings, even with team members who work together daily and regularly, are necessary to remind team members of the values, norms of conduct, and practical procedural plan for every case. There are no shortcuts to achieving this understanding. It requires a robust briefing process by engaged leaders and team members.

Most agree that the time when the briefing process is truly useful is during critical events, when the patient is most in danger of harm. Extraordinary in this common insight is the lack of understanding that, to be performed well in critical situations, actions must be routine, commonplace, and performed excellently during the many rote and straightforward procedures done daily in operating locations. This same logic applies specifically to anesthesia in remote locations.

Anesthesia departments can and should set standards for briefings in remote locations and should require that every case involving anesthesia participation in these areas begin with a briefing. Whether the leader of the briefing is the anesthesia provider or the specialist is open for discussion, depending the experience of the specialty group in performing all the components of a good briefing. These decisions may be based on the size of the provider groups who bring their care to the remote locations and the effort entailed to train the group. In many cases, the anesthesia department may have an easier time training its own members, as long as they then establish the expected norms of conduct for any procedure done in a remote location. The end result will be greater participation in team practice, a greater likelihood that all know the plan for the procedure, and, when combined with effective debriefings, a robust environment for continuous learning.

COMMUNICATION

Three simple communication techniques increase the likelihood that information will be transmitted and received accurately and in a timely fashion. Closing the loop, also known as "read-back" or "hear-back," is the simple technique of repeating back verbally what is requested or described in a manner that assures accurate comprehension. In technical conversations, the process is simple. "I need furosemide, 10 mg, please," would receive a response of "Furosemide, 10 mg." Note that the hear-back in this case does not have to include a "thank you" or any other reflexive social response. The agreed-upon norm of conduct is a succinct repeat back devoid of extraneous words. Closing the loop in this way requires other agreed-upon norms. For example, a request by a surgeon to a surgical technician for a particular instrument may require no verbal response if the placement of the instrument in the appropriate place (eg, the specialist hand) is obvious. Unusual requests, however, always should have a closing of the loop to ensure mutual understanding.

Closing the loop is equally important in complex descriptions such as the history of a patient during a handoff or when a specialist in a remote location is describing a patient and procedure to an anesthesiologist. Closing the loop entails a brief read-back of the information imparted to ensure the anesthesiologist understands what has been described.

Situation, Background, Assessment, Recommendation

A second communication form that promotes critical thinking and frames actions to be taken is a structured communication called "SBAR," an acronym for "situation, background, assessment, and recommendation." In departments where SBAR is used extensively, individuals can frame the conversation by saying, "I'm going to give you an SBAR," thereby telegraphing to the recipient the order of the information about to be imparted. The situation is exactly equivalent to the headline in a newspaper. It should be designed to be brief, succinct, and to capture the attention of the recipient. In a crisis situation, "The situation is that the patient's blood pressure dropped precipitously to 70 mm Hg" is an example of a clear and concerning situation statement.

Background follows in which slightly more expansive information is given to explain the situation. "The blood pressure changed when you cranked open the abdomen and tucked the liver retractor further into position."

Assessment is the evaluation or critical thinking part and is one of SBAR's strengths, in that it promotes the analysis of contributing and causative factors that may help all team members focus on the problem at hand. "I think the extra retraction may be decreasing venous return. Otherwise there's bleeding going on somewhere. If not that, I don't know the problem, but I'm concerned." In and of itself, the concern is enough to warrant the discussion and is a reasonable assessment if a team member's gut feeling is the only precipitant for the SBAR.

The recommendation further drives critical thinking: "Please release the retractor, and let's see where we are." The surgeon may know or see something that the anesthesiologist does not and at this point add or alter the suggested actions. Whatever actions are taken, the SBAR format clarifies for all a structured process of thinking and information sharing. When done well it also promotes learning.

Critical Language

The third communication technique is critical language, an agreed-upon phrase that stops activity, described in other industries as "stopping the line." When a team member perceives a risk and believes that there is limited time to address it, a critical phrase is a useful and powerful mechanism to gain the attention of all team members and momentarily stop all activity. Many obstetric units now use the term, "I need clarity" as the critical statement, known to all team members; its use stops activity so that a group evaluation may be made of the perceived risk. In the obstetrics setting, where every patient is alert and aware and families are often in attendance, the term is neutral and avoids causing unnecessary alarm.

The test of effective teams and leaders occurs not only when the concern is real, because then action is obvious and the team member who picked up the problem is congratulated, but when the concern is inaccurate. The response by other team members determines the health of the team and whether the environment will be a learning, supportive and reliable one in the future. Intolerance of team members when they speak up and are wrong is a sure mechanism to decrease the likelihood of their speaking up in the future.

This practice should not be misconstrued as a requirement to tolerate mediocrity. If an individual repeatedly misunderstands or misrepresents a situation, it is entirely possible that the person needs remediation or is in the wrong position. Well-functioning teams are cognizant of the difference between excellent evaluation of concerns that sometimes are wrong and incompetent evaluations that slow the team from doing its work. As long as the actions taken are appropriate and openly discussed, the environment for outstanding team practice remains viable.

SITUATION AWARENESS AND CONFLICT RESOLUTION

Conflict is an intrinsic part of teamwork. A team's synergy derives from the inputs of each team member and the combining of perspectives and efforts to produce a sum greater than the individual parts. The strength of the team comes from the ability to evaluate, reconcile, combine, and mesh these perspectives into a viewpoint that utilizes the best of all. Along the way, it is likely that team members occasionally will feel strongly and differently and with find themselves in conflict about the team's plan for a procedure. Much of the time these differences are grist for great relationships, and team members probably will appreciate the reconciliation process, because it often is educational. Occasionally differences of opinion flare into disagreement, and the glue of the team membership is tested. At these times hierarchy or strength of personality may determine the course of action rather than what is in the patient's best interest.

Formalized practices to manage conflict can help ensure that the best course of action prevails. An adage that is helpful is "the sun never sets on a disagreement between two team members." In other words, the department(s) should have a codified mechanism for conflict resolution, with all team members committing as a regular and required course of daily action to sit down with those with whom they are in disagreement to resolve the issues. This situation is a true test of leadership, because many of the serious discussions in this setting are unlikely to be successful if left solely to the team members who disagreed. The presence of a moderator—a leader with the formal authority and the informal respect to facilitate a discussion that leads to resolution or "clearing of the air"—often is necessary.

Norms of conduct about challenging team members can help in this regard, and rules of engagement can be agreed upon as a departmental or organizational expectation. Members of the department must agree to abide by these constructs, and department leaders must be willing to censure those who do not follow them. An important part of making these conduct norms real is gaining open commitment by all department members that they will abide by them. This agreement may entail public commitment in departmental meetings and the signing of a document that describes the norms of conduct.

One approach that has shown promise as a mechanism to resolve disagreements is a set of escalating challenges that, if they do not resolve the differences, lead to collaboration with others. One set is to use the words "curious," "concerned," "challenge," and "collaborate." A team member who is troubled by a course of action taken by another team member might say, "I'm curious why you've chosen this particular course of action." In departments where the challenge rules are understood, the recipient would realize that the team member addressing him or her has started a challenge process. If the response does not satisfy the team member's curiosity, the next statement might be, "I'm concerned about the course of action we're taking." This statement ups the ante in the challenge, and the recipient now should appreciate clearly that a negotiation must take place if a further challenge is to be avoided. If the response does not alleviate the concern, the team member may move up to the third level of challenge and say, "I'm not comfortable with this course of action, and I feel I have to challenge it." If circumstances permit, this challenge should lead to a set of prescribed actions, the primary one being involving a third party with the expertise or objectivity to help resolve the difference of opinion. It may be necessary to identify who these arbiters will be, although in some groups it may be adequate that any other member of the team be called upon to help.

The department would have to agree upon a mechanism to help the two team members resolve their differences should an arbiter be unavailable. In some, it is hoped infrequent, situations, a decision will need to be made rapidly or when no third person is available (eg, during middle-of-the-night emergency procedures). In that case, hierarchy and/or accountability for the patient may have to be the deciding factors, although departments might experiment with other, better solutions (eg, a senior person is assigned responsibility for clinical and challenge situations, with the clear understanding that the threshold for calling the arbiter is to be set at a very low level).

No solution covers every situation, but a formal and clear set of conduct norms pertaining to conflict resolution is essential to ensure that the inevitable deviation of behavior from norms that is a characteristic of humans is managed effectively.

LEADERS ENGAGED IN SAFETY AND RELIABILITY THROUGH THE USE OF DATA

The components of team practice that support safe and reliable care require leadership engagement before implementation. Giving an anesthetic in remote locations requires that anesthesia and departmental leadership meet, that the anesthesia leadership understand the concepts described in this article well enough to explain them to others, and that the leaders believe that these concepts are important enough to make them foundational to further action.

Assuming that there is agreement to move forward, education and practice are necessary if the team practices described here are to flourish and be useful. Without ongoing effort, including practice, measurement, and continuous learning, the practices described in this article are likely to extinguish, even in those departments that believe them to be of intrinsic value. They consume some time, and they require the continuous use of a paradigm different from that current in health care today and a kind of reflection that many individuals avoid for many complex reasons. Team excellence requires organizational and individual concentration.

SUMMARY

For many reasons, health care overall has been slow to adopt the reliability engineering well known for decades to other industries. National health care systems have their own reasons, and in each one there are confounders that blind leadership and physicians to many of the threads listed. In the United States the primary problem is in the methods of reimbursement, because payment has been unrelated to quality or safety.

Although prescient leaders are moving forward, there are many pockets of resistance, and significant parts of the United States health system have not started down this path. The general trend, however, is likely to favor those who adapt to the new paradigm, because outcomes now are measurable, benchmarking increasingly is associated with pay for performance, and increasingly well coordinated consumerism will favor the well-organized and forward thinking groups.

The movement of anesthesiologists out of operating rooms is not simply a result of more specialty-specific procedures; it is the result of increasingly precise treatments being performed as part of increasingly prescriptive protocols that, when performed well, achieve targeted and reliable results. The change in anesthesia practice also is a result of the industrialization of health care. These changes can lead to greater levels of reliability if the appropriate factors are considered and managed.

Anesthesia in remote locations depends on the interplay between the anesthesia department and a remote and inevitably complex unit. From an engineering perspective preoccupied with reliability and safety, it is extraordinary how departments of anesthesiology, radiology, gastroenterology, and others expect anesthesiologists to perform effectively in these environments after a brief organizing meeting and without having a constant evaluation of the activity. Concerted and careful planning and evaluation that incorporates the new insights about safety and teamwork will facilitate a level of reliability reassuring to patients and satisfying to clinicians.

REFERENCES

1. Eichhorn JH, Cooper JB, Cullen DJ, et al. Anesthesia practice standards at Harvard: a review. J Clin Anesth 1988;1:55–65.
2. Spear SJ. Learning to lead at Toyota. Harv Bus Rev 2004;82:78–86, 151.
3. Reason JT. Managing the risks of organizational accidents. Brookfield (VT): Ashgate Publishing; 1997.
4. Marx D. Patient safety and the "just culture": a primer for health care executives. New York: Columbia University; 2001.

5. Marx D. How building a "just culture" helps an organization learn from errors. OR Manager 2003;19(1):14–5, 20.
6. Ascension Health Mission Statement. Available at: http://www.ascensionhealth. org/ht_safe/main.asp. Accessed January 5, 2009.
7. Berry LL, Selman KD. Management lessons from Mayo Clinic: inside one of the world's most admired service organizations. New York: McGraw Hill; 2008.

Critical Monitoring Issues Outside the Operating Room

Samuel M. Galvagno, DO[a], Bhavani-Shankar Kodali, MD[b],*

KEYWORDS

- Out of operating room • Pulse oximetry
- Capnography • Monitoring • Anesthesia

Tremendous strides are evident in the nonsurgical interventional care delivered to patients outside of the operating rooms. In the past, both surgical and nonsurgical procedures were performed on sick patients primarily in the operating room (OR). However, recent technologic advances have facilitated the performance of a variety of procedures on complex patients outside of the OR. Many conditions that formerly required surgical intervention are now amenable to noninvasive treatment in interventional suites throughout the hospital.

Unfortunately, however, the physiological monitoring standards for patients undergoing these sophisticated procedures outside of the OR have not evolved concomitantly, and often they are below the standards of care being provided in the OR environment. The reasons for this disparity are that anesthesiologists are not involved in all aspects of care outside of the operating room (OOR), they may not be included in the initial planning stages of the OOR projects, and medical proceduralists are unfamiliar with the monitoring standards that are mandatory within the OR environment for similar procedures.

Improved standards of care in the OR have resulted in a remarkable decrease in morbidity and mortality in the last few decades, which is reflected by the significant decrease in the malpractice premiums of anesthesiologists. To ensure a safe environment for all patients, there is an urgent need to set forth and implement monitoring standards for the procedures performed outside of the ORs and to bring them into alignment with those of ORs. This is particularly necessary for patients with multiple comorbidities and will be increasingly important as non-OR procedures increase in complexity. Although definitive data are lacking, some findings have suggested that adverse events occurring during procedures performed outside of the OR environment have a higher severity of injury and may result from substandard care, including

[a] Johns Hopkins University School of Medicine, Baltimore, MD 21287, USA
[b] Department of Anesthesiology, Perioperative, and Pain Medicine, Brigham and Women's Hospital, Harvard Medical School, Boston, MA 0115, USA
* Corresponding author.
E-mail address: bkodali@partners.org (B-S. Kodali).

Anesthesiology Clin 27 (2009) 141–156
doi:10.1016/j.anclin.2008.11.001
1932-2275/08/$ – see front matter © 2009 Elsevier Inc. All rights reserved.

lack of adherence to minimum monitoring guidelines.[1] This review focuses on the physics, physiology, limitations, and recommendations for standard physiological monitors that should be used in the non-OR environment.

There are three important systems that should be monitored whenever procedures are performed in the OOR setting. They include circulation, ventilation, and oxygenation. Monitors to assess circulation are more often used and familiar to OOR personnel. OOR personnel are also familiar with pulse oximetry. However, OOR personnel are less familiar and often do not monitor ventilation and rely heavily on pulse oximetry as an indirect measure of ventilation. This is inadequate and unsafe. Anesthesiologists must impress upon their medical colleagues the difference between ventilation and oxygenation. Although apnea or hypoventilation usually precedes hypoxemia, the ensuing hypoxia is prevented easily if ventilation is directly monitored. Recognition of hypoventilation or apnea early will provide sufficient time to take corrective action before hypoxemia sets in. The value of capnography as a monitor of ventilation is highlighted in this review.

MONITORS
Pulse Oximetry

Many studies discovered significant knowledge deficits among clinicians regarding the limitations and interpretation of pulse oximetry results.[1-5] An understanding of pulse oximetry is obligatory for all proceduralists and nonanesthesiologists who provide non-OR care, because this technology is used as the principle means of assuring adequate oxygenation in a sedated or anesthetized patient.

Pulse oximetry relies on the spectral analysis of oxygenated and reduced hemoglobin and uses the principle of the Beer-Lambert law.[6-8] This law describes how the concentration of a substance in solution can be determined by transmitting a known intensity of light through a solution. With pulse oximetry, the oxygen saturation (SpO_2) is approximated by transmitting light of a specific wavelength across tissue and measuring its intensity on the other side. Red and near-infrared light readily penetrate tissue, whereas other wavelengths of light tend to be absorbed (**Fig. 1**).

Light-emitting diodes are used to emit red light (660 nm) and near-infrared light (940 nm), because these two wavelengths have known absorption qualities when directed

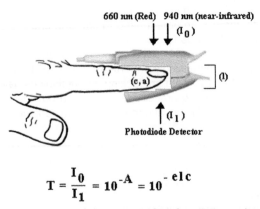

$$T = \frac{I_0}{I_1} = 10^{-A} = 10^{-elc}$$

Fig. 1. Pulse oximetry: Application of the Beer-Lambert law. T, Transmittance; I_0, Intensity of incident light; I_1, Intensity of light after passing through material; A, Absorbance of smaple; I, Distance the light travels; a, Absorption coefficient of the absorber; e, Molar absorptivity of the absorber; c, Concentration of the absorbing species

at hemoglobin (Hb). Specifically, 660-nm red light is absorbed by reduced Hb, whereas 940 nm is absorbed preferentially by oxygenated Hb. When these wavelengths are emitted through tissue and a vascular bed such as a finger, nostril, or earlobe, a photodiode detector on the opposite side measures the amount of light transmitted. The red/near-infrared ratio is calculated by the oximeter and compared with reference values for SpO_2 derived from healthy human subjects. The SpO_2 is further discriminated from venous blood or connective tissue by measuring the pulse-added component of the signal. This signal is comprised of alternating current, representing pulsatile arterial blood, and direct current, which corresponds to tissue, venous blood, and nonpulsatile arterial blood.[9] By canceling out the static components, the pulsatile component can be isolated and the SpO_2 estimated.

Pulse oximetry has several limitations. Nail polish and dark skin may cause a variable degree of interference; the physical obstruction to light transmittance appears to be related to darker skin pigmentation and dark-opaque nail polish.[10–12] In critically ill patients, a low signal-to-noise ratio may exist because of hypovolemia, peripheral vasoconstriction, or peripheral vascular disease.[13] Extra "noise" in the form of ambient light, deflection of light around and not through the vascular bed (optical shunt), and motion artifact may cause false readings.[14–16] Shivering is considered a common source of motion artifact, but normal pulse oximetry readings have been recorded in patients with tonic–clonic seizures.[17]

Dyshemoglobinemias represent a well-known cause of optical interference with pulse oximetry. Both carboxyhemoglobin (COHb) and methemoglobin (MetHb) absorb light within the red and near-infrared wavelength ranges used in pulse oximetry; standard pulse oximeters are unable to distinguish COHb and MetHb from normal oxyhemoglobin (O_2Hb). Hence, COHb will falsely absorb red light, and the pulse oximeter will display a falsely high saturation reading.[18] With MetHb, standard oximeters falsely detect a greater degree of absorption of both Hb and O_2Hb, increasing the absorbance ratio. When the absorbance ratio reaches 1, the calibrated saturation level approaches a plateau of approximately 85%.[19] Co-oximetry offers a multiwavelength analysis that takes into account the absorption of O_2Hb, MetHb, and COHb and should be used to determine an accurate saturation reading in cases in which these dyshemoglobins are suspected. Intravenous dyes such as methylene blue and indigo carmine cause reliable spurious decreases in oximetry readings.[20,21] Fetal hemoglobin, hyperbilirubinemia, and anemia have not been found to yield inaccurate oximetry readings in most cases.[22–24] Newer generations of pulse oximetry have overcome several of these limitations, particularly motion artifact and vasoconstriction. Some units measure carbon monoxide as well as MetHb levels. Measuring MetHb levels have become important with excessive use of benzocaine as local anesthesia for endoscopy procedures. Despite ongoing advances, it is not uncommon to obtain inconsistent waveforms and SpO_2 readings on hemodynamically unstable patients or patients with peripheral vascular disease. When pulse oximetry provides inadequate or unreliable measurements, reliance on monitors of ventilation and circulation becomes critical to ensuring patient well being during procedures.

Capnography

Over the last two decades, capnography has become a standard for monitoring in anesthesia practice.[25] The measurement of carbon dioxide (CO_2) in expired air directly indicates changes in the elimination of CO_2 from the lungs. Indirectly, it indicates changes in the production of CO_2 at the tissue level and in the delivery of CO_2 to the lungs by the circulatory system. Capnography is a noninvasive monitoring technique that allows fast and reliable insight into ventilation, circulation, and metabolism.[26] In the prehospital environment, it is used primarily for confirmation of successful endotracheal intubation, but it may also be a useful indicator of efficient ongoing cardiopulmonary resuscitation. Numerous national organizations, including the American Heart Association, now endorse capnography and capnographic methods for confirming endotracheal tube placement.[27] Despite these recommendations, capnography is not always widely available or consistently applied in the non-OR environment.[28]

Capnometry refers to the measurement and display of CO_2 on a digital or analog monitor. Maximum inspiratory and expiratory CO_2 concentrations during a respiratory cycle are displayed. Capnography refers to the graphic display of instantaneous CO_2 concentration (FCO_2) versus time or expired volume during a respiratory cycle (CO_2 waveform or capnogram). CO_2 waveforms are displayed as two types: FCO_2 versus expired volume (volume capnography) or against time (time capnography). Time capnography is the most common type used in clinical practice.

Infra-red (IR) spectrographs are the most compact and least expensive means to measure end-tidal CO_2 ($ETCO_2$). The wavelength of IR rays exceeds 1.0 millimicrons while the visible spectrum is between 0.4 and 0.8 mμ[29] The IR rays are absorbed by polyatomic gases such as nitrous oxide, CO_2, and water vapor. CO_2 selectively absorbs specific wavelengths (4.3 millimicrons) of IR light (**Fig. 2**). Because the amount of light absorbed is proportional to the concentration of the absorbing molecules, the concentration of a gas can be determined by comparing the measured absorbance with the absorbance of a known standard. The CO_2 concentration measured by the monitor is usually expressed as partial pressure in millimeters of mercury, although some units display percentage CO_2, obtained by dividing the partial pressure of CO_2 by the atmospheric pressure. Other techniques used to measure $ETCO_2$ include Raman spectrography, molecular correlation spectography, mass spectography, and photoacoustic spectography. Infrared technology is cheaper compared with others, and hence is the method of choice used in most capnographs.

A standard terminology for capnography has been adapted.[30] A time capnogram can be divided into inspiratory (phase 0) and expiratory segments (**Fig. 3**). The expiratory segment, similar to a single breath nitrogen curve or single breath CO_2 curve, is divided into three phases (phases I, II, and III). The angle between phase II and phase III is the alpha angle. Alpha angle is an indirect measure of ventilation–perfusion (V/Q) status of the lung. The nearly 90° angle between phase III and the descending limb is the beta angle. Increases in beta angle may indicate presence of rebreathing. The maximal value of expired CO_2 at the end of the expiration is known as end-tidal CO_2 ($ETCO_2$). It can be expressed as percentage CO_2 or, more commonly, as partial pressure in millimeters of mercury ($PETCO_2$). Some causes of increased or decreased $ETCO_2$ are shown in **Box 1**.

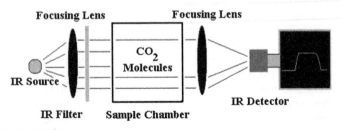

Fig. 2. IR spectrography.

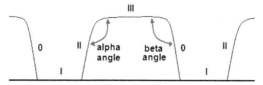

Fig. 3. Current terminology for components of a time capnogram.

Under normal circumstances, the $PETCO_2$ is lower than arterial PCO_2 ($PaCO_2$) by 2 to 5 mm Hg, in adults.[31–34] The PCO_2 gradient is caused by the V/Q mismatch in the lungs as a result of temporal, spatial, and alveolar mixing defects. The arterial-to-end-tidal (a-ET) $PCO_2/PaCO_2$ fraction is a measure of alveolar dead space, and changes in alveolar dead space correlate well with changes in (a-ET) PCO_2.[30] An increase in (a-ET) PCO_2 suggests an increase in dead space ventilation; hence, (a-ET) PCO_2 can provide an indirect estimate of V/Q mismatching of the lung. End-tidal PCO_2 can be used to estimate $PaCO_2$ if there are no abrupt changes in cardiac output or ventilation. However, if there is hemodynamic instability, (a-ET) PCO_2 can vary with varying perfusion to lungs. This changes the ventilation–perfusion relationship, and thereby results in variations in alveolar dead space. Under these circumstances, $PETCO_2$ may not reliably estimate $PaCO_2$.

For a given ventilation, a reduction in cardiac output and pulmonary blood flow results in a decrease in PETCO2 and an increase in (a-ET) PCO_2. Increases in cardiac output and pulmonary blood flow result in better perfusion of the alveoli and an increase in $PETCO_2$.[35] The decrease in (a-ET) PCO_2 is caused by an increase in the alveolar CO_2 suggesting better excretion of CO_2 into the lungs. The improved CO_2 excretion is caused by better perfusion of upper parts of the lung. There is an inverse linear correlation between pulmonary artery pressure and (a-ET) PCO_2.[36] Thus, under conditions of constant lung ventilation, $PETCO_2$ monitoring can be used as a monitor of pulmonary blood flow. Cardiac output and $PETCO_2$ studies have shown good

---

Box 1
Causes of increased or decreased CO_2

Causes of Increased CO_2

Hypoventilation

Hyperthyroidism/Thyroid Storm

Malignant Hyperthermia

Fever/Sepsis

Rebreathing

Other Hypermetabolic States

Causes of Decreased CO_2

Hyperventilation

Hypothermia

Venous Air Embolism

Pulmonary Embolism

Decreased Cardiac Output

Hypoperfusion

correlation between each other. An $ETCO_2$ of 32 mm Hg and 36 mm Hg correlated with a cardiac output 4 L and 5 L, respectively, in intubated and ventilated subjects.

Because of varying (a-ET) PCO_2 in some patients, transcutaneous monitoring of PCO_2 has been used as an alternative to $ETCO_2$ monitoring. In one study of 17 elderly patients, transcutaneous monitoring of PCO_2 provided a more accurate estimation of arterial CO_2 partial pressure than $PETCO_2$ monitoring.[37] At the time of this writing, transcutaneous PCO_2 monitoring is not yet widely available, and the role of this modality for monitoring in the OOR environment has yet to be defined.

End-tidal PCO_2 measurements can also be easily performed in nonintubated spontaneously breathing patients receiving oxygen. However, the resulting waveforms and $PETCO_2$ measurements can be distorted by a dilution effect of air or oxygen resulting in decreased $PETCO_2$ readings. Several varieties of mask and sampling devices are available on the market that provide measurements close to those obtained in intubated patients. Even if the measurements are not quantitatively accurate, they can be considered as baseline measurements/waveforms, and any deviations from baseline during sedation should indicate respiratory depression (see **Figs. 3** and **4**, www.capnography.com, sedation section).

Blood Pressure Measurement

Blood pressure in OOR locations is commonly measured with noninvasive oscillometric devices. An electronic pressure transducer detects oscillating blood flow as the cuff is deflated. Assuming the upper extremity is used, the compressed brachial artery oscillates as restricted blood flows through it and the systolic, diastolic, and mean pressures are determined. An in-depth discussion of invasive intra-arterial techniques

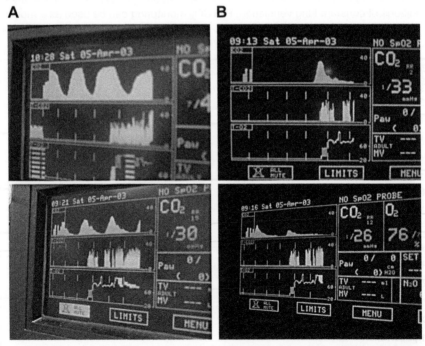

Fig. 4. Examples of oversedation as seen on capnography. (A) Baseline. (B) Oversedation.

is beyond the scope of this article; for further information, an excellent review by Polanco and Pinsky is available.[38]

Electrocardiography

Both transmural and subendocardial ischemia can be detected when electrocardiography (ECG) leads are properly positioned.[39] Lead V_5, the precordial lead originally described in Kaplan and King's classic report on intraoperative ischemia, has been validated and found to detect up to 75% of ischemic changes seen in all 12 leads.[40,41] The combination of leads II, V_2, V_3, V_4, and V_5, has a sensitivity of 100% for detecting intraoperative ischemia.[39] The reader is directed to an exceptional review on perioperative electrocardiography previously published in *Anesthesiology Clinics*.[42]

Temperature Monitoring

Perioperative hypothermia increases the incidence of adverse myocardial outcomes, increases blood loss, and increases wound infection.[43–45] Mild hypothermia also changes the kinetics of various anesthetics and may delay postoperative recovery.[45] Intraoperative hypothermia usually develops in three phases. The first phase is caused by redistribution of heat from the core thermal compartment to the outer shell of the body. A slower, linear reduction in the core temperature follows and may last several hours.[45] In the last phase, the core temperature plateaus and may remain unchanged throughout the remainder of the perioperative period as thermoregulatory control is impaired during general or regional anesthesia. Numerous temperature monitoring devices are available, but it is the site of temperature monitoring rather than the type of temperature probe that is most important. Core temperature can be estimated from accessible sites such as the nasopharynx, bladder, esophageal, or rectal sites.[45] Temperature monitoring has become a standard of care, and anesthesiologists are expected to be proactive in maintaining normothermia and preventing temperature derangements throughout the perioperative period. Most of the OOR environments are kept at lower temperatures to protect the expensive equipment. Therefore, it is essential that temperature monitoring is an integral part of the monitoring systems in OOR.

Spontaneous Electroencephalographic Activity Monitors

Depth of anesthesia monitoring with the bispectral index monitor (BIS) has been shown to reduce, but not eliminate, the incidence of awareness under anesthesia.[46] In the neurocritical care setting, BIS monitoring has been shown to provide a more objective means of sedation assessment that may lead to a decrease in overall rates of propofol administration and fewer incidences of oversedation.[47] A recent Cochrane review concluded that anesthesia guided by BIS within the recommended range (40 to 60) could improve anesthetic delivery and postoperative recovery from relatively deep anesthesia while reducing the incidence of intraoperative recall in surgical patients at a high risk for awareness.[48] The Patient State Index (PSI) is another monitor for awareness that has not been studied as thoroughly as the BIS, but has been shown to provide indications that correlate with unconsciousness.[49] For a detailed review of the current state of monitors for preventing intraoperative awareness, the reader is directed to the American Society of Anesthesiologists' (ASA's) 2006 Practice Advisory.[50]

CONSIDERATIONS FOR MONITORING IN OUT-OF-OR ENVIRONMENTS
The Magnetic Resonance Imaging Suite

Magnetic resonance imaging (MRI) poses a profound risk to patients with implanted ferromagnetic material because the high magnetic field may dislodge pacemakers, implants, cardiac valves, or other prostheses. Before entering the MRI suite, all ferromagnetic items need to be removed from the care provider's possession to prevent injury; an MRI-compatible anesthesia machine and equipment are compulsory.[51] The intense radiofrequency may cause surface heating on the patient's body, and the lead wires from the ECG also pose a potential burn hazard.[52] The ECG monitor is subject to considerable artifact from the background static magnetic field and radiofrequency impulses as well as the electronics within the device that create magnetic fields.[53] Modern devices minimize these limitations and advances in ECG monitoring in the MRI suite continue. Blood pressure monitoring by the oscillometric method is most commonly used and provides reliable readings. Pulse oximetry may be difficult in the MRI suite because the signal may become degraded as a result of currents in the oximetry cable and a decreased signal-to-noise ratio.[54] A decrease in the phase II slope of the capnogram may be observed because of a long circuit pathway. Remote monitoring via a closed-circuit monitor—preferably with zoom lens magnification capability—may be necessary. Several MRI-compatible monitors measure cardiovascular, ventilatory (capnography), and oxygenation (pulse oximetry) reliably, and, therefore, all patients undergoing MRI can be monitored as they would be in the OR.

Computed Tomography

An anesthetized patient in the computed tomography (CT) scanner presents logistical problems similar to those encountered in the MRI suite; however, the impact on interference with standard monitors is not as profound. Blood pressure should be monitored at relatively short intervals because radiocontrast media reactions may lead to a precipitous loss of systemic vascular resistance. Standard monitors such as the ECG, temperature probe, pulse oximetry, and capnography should be used. As with procedures done in the MRI suite and elsewhere, remote monitoring may be required. Frequently, apnea is requested during fluoroscopy, and capnography is essential to serve as a reminder to start the ventilator if forgotten inadvertently.

Electroconvulsive Therapy

Electroconvulsive therapy (ECT) is used for treatment of severe psychiatric disorders as well as depression, complex regional pain syndrome, and chronic pain.[55] ECT involves provocation of a generalized epileptic seizure by electrical stimulation of the brain. The procedure usually is preformed under general anesthesia with muscle relaxation. Excessive alterations in heart rate, blood pressure, and cardiac functions are prevented by anticholinergic and antihypertensive agents; hence, blood pressure and ECG monitoring is mandatory.[56] Train-of-four monitoring for neuromuscular blockade and BIS monitoring should also be considered. Capnography is essential for safe and effective anesthetic management of patients undergoing ECT, especially patients with intracranial disorders or coronary artery disease.[57]

The Endoscopy Suite

Most endoscopic procedures are performed in an OOR environment, and in many cases, these procedures may be accomplished with moderate or deep sedation. Capnography should be used because significant delays in detecting respiratory compromise have been shown in its absence.[58] In addition to blood pressure and ECG monitoring, pulse oximetry and capnography should be considered standard monitors to ensure adequate ventilation and oxygenation during endoscopic procedures, whether they be performed under general anesthesia or varying degrees of sedation.[59] The American Society of Gastrointestinal Endoscopy and the British Society of Gastroenterology issue guidelines periodically to impress upon practitioners the need to be proactive in detecting and eliminating hypoxia during gastrointestinal procedures.

Interventional Angiography

ECG, blood pressure, pulse oximetry, and capnography are standard monitors for procedures in interventional angiography. In addition, intracranial pressure monitoring (ICP) and invasive arterial blood pressure monitoring are frequently used. In some instances, central venous pressure monitoring and monitoring of evoked potentials may be necessary. In recent years, the endovascular treatment of diseases of intracranial and spinal vessels has become widely accepted; invasive monitoring is frequently required based on the usual underlying pathophysiology and severity of these disorders.[60]

Controversies in monitoring

Numerous investigators have focused in the ability of monitors to prevent morbidity and mortality. In a well-known randomized, controlled trial by Watkinson and colleagues,[61] the investigators concluded that mandated electronic vital signs monitoring in high-risk medical and surgical patients had no effect on adverse events or mortality. Although this study had numerous limitations that may have led to type II error, the "number needed to monitor" to alter outcomes was estimated to be large.[61] In a systematic review of randomized, controlled trials examining the role of pulse oximetry, there was no evidence of a significant difference between groups regarding duration of postoperative mechanical ventilation, duration of intensive care unit stay, or postoperative complications; the investigators were unable to find reliable evidence that pulse oximetry affects the outcome of anesthesia.[62] Moller's landmark studies in 1993, based on a design that was similar to both a randomized, controlled trial and a cluster randomized trial that included 20,802 patients, concluded that pulse oximetry did not have a significant impact on mortality or hospital stay.[63–65] In a review of clinical trials on monitoring, the authors acknowledge that pulse oximetry may enable clinicians to detect desaturation episodes more readily and that this technology may be beneficial, but to prevent one adverse event, a large number of patients must be monitored.[66] The findings of these and other related studies were summarized in a Cochrane review that concluded that the value of perioperative monitoring with pulse oximetry is unproven.[67]

Earlier studies, including a closed claims analysis, suggested that pulse oximetry was an invaluable modality for preventing adverse outcomes in anesthesia, and that improvements in monitoring—specifically pulse oximetry—may have helped reduce serious mishaps over the last several decades by at least 35%.[68] Two additional studies suggested that monitoring with pulse oximetry facilitates early detection of arterial hypoxemia, allowing earlier and potentially life-saving treatment.[65,69] Oversedation with ensuing respiratory depression is an important contributor to adverse events that have occurred under monitored anesthesia care, and appropriate use of monitoring has been cited as a crucial preventative measure that often is neglected.[70] Studies based on analyses of closed claims data suggest that better monitoring may lead to earlier correction of potentially harmful perioperative events.[71,72]

Despite numerous national guidelines and recommendations, there seems to be a paucity of data to support the use of monitors in preventing mortality outside of the OR. In 2006, Watkinson and colleagues[61] studied 402 heterogeneous high-risk medical and surgical ward patients, and failed to demonstrate that monitoring heart rate, noninvasive blood pressure, oxygen saturation, respiratory rate by impedance pneumography, and skin temperature could predict or identify adverse outcomes. Similarly, when a medical emergency team was tasked with closely following vital signs in an effort to rapidly recognize critical threshold patterns suggestive of potential adverse events, no benefit was found.[73] Although each of these studies had significant limitations, they helped promulgate the idea that mandatory monitoring, even with a high incidence of abnormal vital signs, does not confer a mortality benefit. Nevertheless, other investigators determined that improved monitoring might have prevented a significant number of adverse outcomes identified in the ASA closed claims database.[74]

Initial studies using capnography as a supplement during procedures requiring sedation suggested that this practice might serve as an early warning mechanism for impending respiratory embarrassment.[75,76] Capnography may have an advantage over pulse oximetry because capnography is a better measure of ventilation. With capnography, providers are able to institute early stimulation for nonbreathing patients, thereby preventing arterial oxygen desaturation. Lightdale and colleagues[77] found that microstream capnography significantly prevented arterial oxygen desaturation in children undergoing sedation for procedures. This was an important finding because most of the calamitous events during sedation occur secondarily to hypoventilation and respiratory failure.[78]

The zone between sedation and anesthesia is very narrow. When the patient drifts away from conscious sedation to a state in which there is no response to verbal commands or sensory stimuli, he approaches general anesthesia. The width of this safety zone depends on the physical condition of the patient, amount of sedatives used, potency of medications, and stimulation arising from the procedure. When the stimulation suddenly ceases, this can induce a relative excess of sedation leading to hypoventilation or apnea. If not readily detected and corrected, this can culminate in hypoxemia. Sometimes, visual observation of patient is not possible, either because of the type of procedure or dark rooms that are necessary for good visualization of LCD screens by the interventionists performing noninvasive procedures. Therefore, it is likely that every patient being given so-called "conscious sedation," at some time or the other during the course of the sedation procedure, will drift into a state of deep sedation or general anesthesia. The duration of this depends on the factors enumerated above. Hence, it can be logically argued that any patient receiving sedation also qualifies for ASA standards of monitoring and should have their circulatory, ventilatory, and oxygenation status monitored in standard fashion. Ironically, administration of supplementary oxygen to the patients compounds the problem further. The goal of supplemental oxygen is to increase oxygen reserves, thereby delaying or preventing the onset of hypoxia. It has been shown that super oxygenated patients desaturate only after prolonged apnea.[79,80] This negates the use of pulse oximetry as an early warning monitoring device for respiratory depression, which is concerning in light of the fact that the majority of sedation providers rarely recognize respiratory depression in sedated patients who do not become hypoxic.[81] In one study, the treating physicians blinded to capnography could not identify apneic episodes during sedation procedures.[82] In the same study, absolute $ETCO_2$ change of greater than 10 mm Hg identified nine of 25 patients who experienced hypoxia (36% sensitive) (95% confidence interval [CI], 18% to 57%) and 68% specific (95% CI, 57% to 77%); positive predictive value (PPV), 32%; negative predictive value (NPPV), 67%. An absolute $ETCO_2$ change from baseline of greater than 10% would have identified 18 of the 25 patients before hypoxia developed (sensitivity, 72% [95% CI, 59% to 93%]; specificity, 47% [95% CI, 36% to 58%]; PPV, 37%; NPV, 80%).

RECOMMENDATIONS

Although data to support a mortality benefit appear to be lacking, numerous organizations, including the ASA, strongly endorse monitoring in OOR environments.[83,84] A letter in the *British Medical Journal* was concerned about the relatively higher death rate of 1 in 2000 from upper gastrointestinal endoscopy, which is usually performed under sedation or local anesthesia, or both,[85] compared with the overall morality solely attributable to anesthesia, which is 1 in 185,000 or higher. The OR environment has become safer because of stringent monitoring standards. There is an urgent need to take proactive measures and follow a set of standard guidelines to enhance the safety of patients undergoing OOR procedures. It is only a matter of time before medico-legal scenarios will shift to OOR locations, where more patients will be cared for, and inadequate monitoring may contribute to morbidity and mortality. For OOR anesthetizing locations, the ASA recommends that the Standards for Basic Anesthetic Monitoring (**Table 1**) be followed.[86]

In a busy hospital practice, it is not uncommon to hear "code blue" being called from OOR locations. The majority of these emergencies are ventilation-related incidents that occur during procedural sedation performed by nonanesthesiologists. If anesthesiologists provide sedation, capnography typically is used in addition to other monitors, as recommended by ASA. When sedation is administered by nonanesthesia personnel, we strongly recommend that ventilation be monitored during all procedures (**Table 2**). There is ongoing educational process in our institution to train nonanesthesia personnel in the value of capnography as a ventilation monitor. At the moment, capnography seems to be the best available device for ventilatory monitoring. Hence, it is the onus of physicians overseeing sedation procedures to encourage the monitoring ventilation to increase the safety of the patients under their care.

Table 1	
Standards for basic anesthetic monitoring	
Parameter	**Methods**
Equipment	Anesthesia equipment, machine should be set up in standard format identical to OR to minimize unfamiliarity to the anesthesiologists.
Oxygenation	Inspired gas oxygen analyzer pulse oximetry (with audible tone). Illumination to assess the patient's color.
Ventilation	$PETCO_2$ monitoring: Capnography with audible CO_2 alarm to detect correct placement of endotracheal tube. Use of a device capable of detecting disconnection of the components of the breathing system. Detection of hypoventilation.
Circulation	Continuous electrocardiogram blood pressure and heart rate determination no less than every 5 minutes. Assessment by at least one of the following: palpation of a pulse, intra-arterial tracing of blood pressure, ultrasound peripheral pulse monitoring, pulse plethysmography, or oximetry.
Body Temperature	Indicated when clinical significant changes in body temperature are intended, anticipated, or suspected.

Table 2
Recommended monitoring for procedural sedation

Parameter	Methods
Training	Physicians must understand the value of monitoring and undergo procedural sedation course.
Establishment of protocols	All the OOR sites should have uniform protocols so that their implementation is easy and uniform across all sites.
Oxygenation	Pulse oximetry (with audible tone). Illumination to assess the patient's color.
Ventilation	PETCO$_2$ monitoring: Capnography with audible CO$_2$ alarm to detect hypoventilation and apnea.
Circulation	Continuous electrocardiogram. Blood pressure and heart rate determination no less than every 5 minutes.
Body Temperature	Indicated when clinical significant changes in body temperature are expected during long noninvasive procedures.
Review protocols	Periodic review of problems encountered and appropriate amendments made to protocols to ensure that the problems do not recur.

SUMMARY

Monitoring standards in OOR locations should not differ from those in the OR. Because of extraordinary developments in medical, surgical, and radiologic techniques, sicker patients are being cared for outside of traditional ORs. It is essential that we keep pace with these evolving changes and make improvements needed to provide the same standard of monitoring care outside of the OR as we rely on in the ORs. Furthermore, some of the OOR locations are remote from main operating locations, and it may take considerable time to respond to any emergencies and codes that may arise in these locations. Although the true rate of complications from anesthesia in the OOR environment is currently unknown, we should not wait to implement standards for monitoring until disasters occur. There is no need to reinvent the wheel to determine the need for vigilant monitoring in OOR settings. Anesthesiologists have evolved a robust system of monitoring standards based on decades of experience in OR environments. Every OOR location should be thoroughly evaluated with monitoring standards implemented. These standards should be periodically reviewed to avert morbidity.

REFERENCES

1. Robbertze R, Posner K, Domino K. Closed claims review of anesthesia for procedures outside the operating room. Curr Opin Anaesthesiol 2006;19:436–42.
2. Sinex J. Pulse oximetry: principles and limitations. Am J Emerg Med 1999;17: 59–67.
3. Elliott M, Tate R, Page K. Do clinicians know how to use pulse oximetry? A literature review and clinical implications. Aust Crit Care 2006;19:139–44.
4. Rodriguez L, Kotin N, Lowenthal D, et al. A study of pediatric house staff's knowledge of pulse oximetry. Pediatrics 1994;93:810–3.
5. Stoneham M, Saville G, Wilson I. Knowledge about pulse oximetry among medical and nursing staff. Lancet 1994;344:1339–42.

6. Kelleher J. Pulse oximetry. J Clin Monit 1989;5:37–62.
7. Tremper K, Barker S. Pulse oximetry. Anesthesiology 1989;70:98–108.
8. Salyer J. Neonatal and pediatric pulse oximetry. Respir Care 2003;48:386–96.
9. Wukitsch M, Petterson M, Tobler DR, et al. Pulse oximetry: analysis of theory, technology, and practice. J Clin Monit 1988;4:290–301.
10. Volgyesi G, Spahr-Schopfer I. Does skin pigmentation affect the accuracy of pulse oximetry? An in vitro study. Anesthesiology 1991;75:A406.
11. Cote C, Goldsteing E, Fuchsman W, et al. The effect of nail polish on pulse oximetry. Anesth Analg 1988;67:683–6.
12. Ries A, Prewitt L, Johnson J. Skin color and ear oximetry. Chest 1989;96:287–90.
13. Severinghaus J, Spellman M. Pulse oximeter failure thresholds in hypotension and vasoconstriction. Anesthesiology 1990;73:532–7.
14. Hanowell L, Eisele JH, Downs D. Ambient light affects pulse oximeters. Anesthesiology 1987;67:864–5.
15. Costarino A, Davis D, Keon T. Falsely normal saturation reading with the pulse oximeter. Anesthesiology 1987;67:830–1.
16. Severinghaus JW, Kelleher JF. Recent developments in pulse oximetry. Anesthesiology 1992;76(6):1018–38.
17. James M, Marshall H, Carew-McColl M. Pulse oximetry during apparent tonic-clonic seizures. Lancet 1991;337:394–5.
18. Buckley R, Aks S, Eshom J, et al. The pulse oximetry gap in carbon monoxide intoxication. Ann Emerg Med 1994;24:252–5.
19. Barker S, Tremper KK, Hyatt J. Effects of methemoglobinemia on pulse oximetry and mixed venous oximetry. Anesthesiology 1989;70:112–7.
20. Kessler M, Eide T, Humayan B, et al. Spurious pulse oximeter desaturation with methylene blue injection. Anesthesiology 1986;65:435–6.
21. Scheller M, Unger R, Kelner M. Effects of intravenously administered dyes on pulse oximetry readings. Anesthesiology 1986;65:550–2.
22. Severinghaus J, Koh S. Effect of anemia on pulse oximeter accuracy at low saturation. J Clin Monit 1990;85–8.
23. Harris A, Sendak M, Donham R, et al. Absorption characteristics of human fetal hemoglobin at wavelengths used in pulse oximetry. J Clin Monit 1988;4:175–7.
24. Ramanathan R, Durand M, Larrazabal C. Pulse oximetry in very low birth weight infants with acute and chronic disease. Pediatrics 1987;79(4):612–7.
25. Kodali B, Moseley H, Kumar A, et al. Capnography and anaesthesia: review article. Can J Anaesth 1992;39:617–32.
26. Kupnik D, Skok P. Capnometry in the prehospital setting: are we using its potential? J Emerg Med 2007;24:614–7.
27. American Heart Association. 2005 American heart association guidelines for cardiopulmonary resuscitation and emergency cardiovascular care. Part 7.1: adjuncts for airway control and ventilation. Circulation 2005;112:IV-51–7.
28. Deiorio M. Continuous end-tidal carbon dioxide monitoring for confirmation of endotracheal tube placement is neither widely available nor consistently applied by emergency physicians. J Emerg Med 2005;22:490–3.
29. Colman Y, Krauss B. Microstream capnography technology: a new approach to an old problem. J Clin Monit 1999;15.
30. Kodali B, Kumar A, Moseley H, et al. Terminology and the current limitations of time capnography: A brief review. J Clin Monit 1995;11:175–82.
31. Nunn J, Hill D. Respiratory dead space and arterial to end-tidal CO2 tension difference in anesthetized man. J Appl Phys 1960;15:383–9.

32. Fletcher R, Jonson B. Deadspace and the single breath test carbon dioxide during anaesthesia and artificial ventilation. Br J Anaesth 1984;56:109–19.

33. Kodali B, Moseley H, Kumar Y, et al. Arterial to end-tidal carbon dioxide tension difference during Caesarean section anaesthesia. Anaesthesia 1986;41: 698–702.

34. Fletcher R, Jonson B, Cumming G, et al. The concept of dead space with special reference to the single breath test for carbon dioxide. Br J Anaesth 1981;53: 77–88.

35. Leigh M, Jones J, Motley H. The expired carbon dioxide as a continuous guide of the pulmonary and circulatory systems during anesthesia and surgery. J Thorac Cardiovasc Surg 1961;41:597–610.

36. Askrog V. Changes in (a-A) CO2 difference and pulmonary artery pressure in anesthetized man. J Appl Phys 1966;21:1299–305.

37. Casati A, Squicciarini G, Malagutti G, et al. Transcutaneous monitoring of partial pressure of carbon dioxide in the elderly patient: a prospective, clinical comparison with end-tidal monitoring. J Clin Anesth 2006;18:436–40.

38. Polanco P, Pinsky M. Practical issues of hemodynamic monitoring at the bedside. Surg Clin North Am 2006;86:1431–56.

39. Fuchs R, Achuff S, Grunwald L, et al. Electrocardiographic localization of coronary artery narrowings: studies during myocardial ischemia and infarction in patients with one-vessel disease. Circulation 1982;66:1168–76.

40. Kaplan J, King S. The precordial electrocardiographic lead (V5) in patients who have coronary-artery disease. Anesthesiology 1976;45:570–4.

41. London M, Hollenberg M, Wong W, et al. Intraoperative myocardial ischemia: localization by continuous 12-lead electrocardiography. Anesthesiology 1988; 69:232–41.

42. John A, Fleisher L. Electrocardiography: the ECG. Anesthesiol Clin 2006;24: 697–715.

43. Kurz A, Sessler D, Lenhardt R. Perioperative normothermia to reduce the incidence of surgical-wound infection and shorten hospitalization. Study of wound infection and temperature group. N Engl J Med 1996;334:1209–15.

44. Pestel GJ, Kurz A. Hypothermia—it's more than a toy. Curr Opin Anaesthesiol 2005;18(2):151–6.

45. Insler S, Sessler D. Perioperative thermoregulation and temperature monitoring. Anesthesiol Clin 2006;24:823–37.

46. Bruhn J, Myles P, Sneyd R, et al. Depth of anaesthesia monitoring: what's available, what's validated and what's next? Br J Anaesth 2006;97:85–94.

47. Olson D, Cheek D, Morgenlander J. The impact of bispectral index monitoring on rates of propofol administration. AACN clinical issues: advanced practice in acute & critical care. Biol Med 2004;1:63–73.

48. Punjasawadwong Y, Boonjeungmonkol N, Phongchiewboon A. Bispectral index for improving anaesthetic delivery and postoperative recovery. Cochrane Database Syst Rev 2007;4:CD003843.

49. Chen X, Tang J, White P, et al. A comparison of patient state index and bispectral index values during the perioperative period. Anesth Analg 2002;95: 1669–74.

50. Apfelbaum J, Arens J, Cole D, et al, for the American Society of Anesthesiologists Task Force on Intraoperative Awareness Practice advisory for intraoperative awareness and brain function monitoring. Anesthesiology 2006;104:847–64.

51. Deckert D, Zecha-Stallinger A, Haas T, et al. Anesthesia outside the core operating area. Anaesthesist 2007;56:1028–30, 32–7.

52. Rejger V, Cohn B, Vielvoye G, et al. A simple anaesthetic and monitoring system for magnetic resonance imaging. Eur J Anaesthesiol 1989;6:373–8.

53. Patterson S, Chesney J. Anesthetic management for magnetic resonance imaging: problems and solutions. Anesth Analg 1992;74(1):121–8.

54. Peden CJ, Menon DK, Hall AS, et al. Magnetic resonance for the anaesthetist. Anesthesia 1992;47(6):508–17.

55. Grundmann U, Oest M. Anaesthesiological aspects of electroconvulsive therapy. Anaesthesist 2007;56:202–4, 6–11.

56. Saito S. Anesthesia management for electroconvulsive therapy: hemodynamic and respiratory management. J Anesth 2005;19:142–9.

57. Saito S, Kadoi Y, Nihishara F, et al. End-tidal carbon dioxide monitoring stabilized hemodynamic changes during ECT. J ECT 2003;19:26–30.

58. Pino R. The nature of anesthesia and procedural sedation outside of the operating room. Curr Opin Anaesthesiol 2007;20:347–51.

59. Melloni C. Anesthesia and sedation outside the operating room: how to prevent risk and maintain good quality. Curr Opin Anaesthesiol 2007;20:513–9.

60. Preiss H, Reinartz J, Lowens S, et al. Anesthesiological management of neuroendovascular interventions. Anaesthesist 2006;55:679–92.

61. Watkinson P, Barber V, Price J, et al. A randomised controlled trial of the effect of continuous electronic physiological monitoring on the adverse event rate in high risk medical and surgical patients. Anesthesia 2006;61:1031–9.

62. Pedersen T, Moller AM, Pedersen BD. Pulse oximetry for perioperative monitoring: systematic review of randomized, controlled trials. Anesth Analg 2003;96(2):426–31.

63. Moller J, Johannessen N, Espersen K, et al. Randomized evaluation of pulse oximetry in 20,802 patients: II. Perioperative events and postoperative complications. Anesthesiology 1993;78:445–53.

64. Moller J, Pedersen T, Rasmussen L, et al. Randomized evaluation of pulse oximetry in 20,802 patients: I. Design, demography, pulse oximetry failure rate, and overall complication rate. Anesthesiology 1993;78:436–44.

65. Moller J, Wittrup M, Johansen S. Hypoxemia in the postanesthesia care unit: an observer study. Anesthesiology 1990;73:890–5.

66. Young D, Griffiths J. Clinical trials of monitoring in anaesthesia, critical care and acute ward care: a review. Br J Anaesth 2006;97:39–45.

67. Pedersen T, Pedersen B, Moller A. Pulse oximetry for Perioperative monitoring. Cochrane Database Syst Rev 2003;3:CD002013.

68. Tinker J, Dull D, Caplan R, et al. Role of monitoring devices in prevention of anesthetic mishaps: a closed claims analysis. Anesthesiology 1989;71:541–6.

69. Cote CJ, Rolf N, Liu LM, et al. A single-blind study of combined pulse oximetry and capnography in children. Anesthesiology 1991;74(6):980–7.

70. Bhananker S, Posner K, Cheney F, et al. Injury and liability associated with monitored anesthesia care: a closed claims analysis. Anesthesiology 2006;104:228–34.

71. Cooper J, Cullen D, Nemeskal R, et al. Effects of information feedback and pulse oximetry on the incidence of anesthesia complications. Anesthesiology 1987;67:686–94.

72. Cooper J, Newbower R, Kitz R. An analysis of major errors and equipment failures in anesthesia management: considerations for prevention and detection. Anesthesiology 1984;60:34–42.

73. Hillman K, Chen J, Cretikos M, et al. Introduction of the medical emergency team (MET) system: a cluster-randomized controlled trial. Lancet 2005;365:2091–7.

74. Caplan R, Posner K, Ward R, et al. Adverse respiratory events in anesthesia: a closed claims analysis. Anesthesiology 1990;72:828–33.
75. Soto R, Fu E, Vila H, et al. Capnography accurately detects apnea during monitored anesthesia care. Anesth Analg 2004;99:379–82.
76. Vargo J, Zuccaro G, Dumot J, et al. Automated graphic assessment of respiratory activity is superior to pulse oximetry and visual assessment for the detection of early respiratory depression during therapeutic upper endoscopy. Gastrointest Endosc 2002;55:826–31.
77. Lightdale J, Goldmann D, Feldman H, et al. Microstream capnography improves patient monitoring during moderate sedation: a randomized, controlled trial. Pediatrics 2006;117:e1170–80.
78. Cote C, Notterman D, Karl H. Adverse sedation events in pediatrics: a critical incident analysis of contributing factors. Pediatrics 2000;105:805–14.
79. Jense HG, Dubin SA, Silverstein PI, et al. Effect of obesity on safe duration of apnea in anesthetized humans. Anesth Analg 1991;72:89–93.
80. Patel R, Lenczyk M, Hannallah RS, et al. Age and the onset of desaturation in apnoeic children. Can J Anaesth 1994;41:771–4.
81. Deitch K, Chudnofsky CR, Dominici P. The utility of supplemental oxygen during emergency department procedural sedation and analgesia with midozolam and fentanyl: a randomized, controlled trial. Ann Emerg Med 2007;49:1–8.
82. Deitch K, Chudnofsky CR, Dominici P. The utility of supplemental oxygen during emergency department procedural sedation with propofol: a randomized, controlled trial. Ann Emerg Med 2008;52:1–8.
83. The American Society of Anesthesiologists. Guidelines for nonoperating room anesthetizing locations. 2003. Avaliable at: http://www.asahq.org/publicationsAndServices/standards/14.pdf. Accessed June 23, 2008.
84. Cote C, Wilson S, Sedation and the Workgroup on Sedation. Guidelines for monitoring and management of pediatric patients during and after sedation for diagnostic and therapeutic procedures. Pediatrics 2006;118:2587–602.
85. Appaddurai IR, Delicta RJ, Carey PD, et al. Monitoring during endoscopy. BMJ 1995;311(7002):452.
86. The American Society of Anesthesiologists. Standards for basic anesthetic monitoring. 2005. Avaliable at: http://www.asahq.org/publicationsAndServices/standards/02.pdf. Accessed June 23, 2008.

The Evolution of the Anesthesiologist: Novel Perioperative Roles and Beyond

Richard Teplick, MD[a],*, Myer Rosenthal, MD[b]

KEYWORDS

- Out-of OR anesthesia • Anesthesiology consultants
- Surgical hospitalists • Perioperative care
- Anesthesiology residency training • Critical care
- Anesthesiology fellowships

Delivery of the spectrum of anesthesia from sedation to general anesthesia for patients undergoing procedures outside of the operating room (OR) poses several problems not encountered in the OR. These include limited time to assess the patient and often no time to obtain consultations for medical conditions that may be outside of the usual purview of an anesthesiologist, such as initial management of infections, diabetic ketoacidosis or hyperosmotic hyperglycemic state, inadequately managed cardiovascular disease, and toxic ingestions. Anesthesiologists trained in critical care usually have more experience with the initial assessment and management of patients with such conditions. Some of these conditions, however, also draw on training in internal medicine that is usually not provided in the continuum of anesthesiology residencies or anesthesiology critical care fellowships. Consequently, it can be argued that because procedures performed outside of the OR are becoming more common, the curriculum for anesthesia residencies should be modified to provide more training in conditions typically assessed and managed by internists or medical subspecialists.

Many anesthesiologists have written about expanding anesthesia into the perioperative arena, usually referring not only to increasing the role of anesthesiologists in the already established programs in pain management and critical care but also expanding into the relatively less formalized roles in the preoperative and postoperative assessment and in-hospital management of surgical patients.[1-9] One arena that has received relatively little attention is the increasing number and complexity of patients undergoing procedures outside of the OR who often have multiple medical problems,

[a] University of South Alabama Hospitals, University of South Alabama College of Medicine, 2451 Fillingim Street, University of South Alabama Medical Center, Mobile, AL 36617, USA
[b] Department of Anesthesiology, Stanford University, CA, USA
* Corresponding author.
E-mail address: teplick@zeus.bwh.harvard.edu (R. Teplick).

Anesthesiology Clin 27 (2009) 157–165
doi:10.1016/j.anclin.2009.01.004
1932-2275/09/$ – see front matter © 2009 Elsevier Inc. All rights reserved.

yet are frequently seen by an anesthesiologist for the first time just before their procedure. Such patients pose a unique and difficult challenge not only because of the logistics in providing personnel and equipment for such services but also in needing rapid assimilation and adaptation to such patients' medical needs. Just as in the OR, knowledge of anesthesia and the procedure to be performed are essential for out-of-OR anesthesia or sedation. In addition, the anesthesiologist needs to be able to assess the patient's medical comorbidities and rapidly adjust the anesthetic plan and management to minimize the risks these conditions impose. This frequently must be done just before the procedure is to begin without any prior anesthetic evaluation of the patient and without the resources and personnel available in the OR. Because there is usually insufficient time to obtain consultations, patient assessment often falls solely on the anesthesiologist.

The actual implementation of the anesthetic plan during out-of-OR anesthesia or sedation for patients with serious medical problems requires considerable skill. It does not, however, necessarily require understanding the potential interactions of a patient's comorbidities with the risks of both the procedure and the drugs needed for anesthesia or sedation if the anesthetic plan and oversight is provided by someone who appreciates these issues. Such supervision requires a combination of both the knowledge and experience gained during general medicine training and the experience and understanding of the mechanics of anesthesia and the drugs used in its delivery gained during a residency in anesthesiology.[10] The requisite general medical knowledge and experience are similar to but often more extensive than that required in many of the perioperative fields in which anesthesiologists currently participate, as well as that acquired during the base year and anesthesia residency. However, this combination of skills and knowledge is easily within reach of anesthesiologists with some additional training in general medicine but outside the scope of knowledge and familiarity of internists without anesthesia training. For anesthesiologists successfully to continue the foray into perioperative medicine, including out-of-OR anesthesia, anesthesia training must change to include more general medicine and an increasing emphasis on consultation and supervision rather than the hands-on delivery of anesthesia. Specifically, the major role of the anesthesiologist should shift to that of a consultant delineating the anesthetic considerations and plan; perhaps not actually providing the anesthesia but rather guiding the delivery by skilled nonphysician practitioners.

During the deliberation of the American Society of Anesthesiologists Taskforce on Future Paradigms of Anesthesia Practice in 2004 and 2005, it became quite evident that a "value-added" approach to anesthesia practice must be considered if anesthesiology is to survive as a respected and vital contributing medical specialty. In a special 2005 supplement to *The Hospitalist*, the official publication of the Society of Hospital Medicine, the belief that internal medicine provides the best opportunity and training for surgical perioperative care was clearly expressed. In the opening editorial, Geno Merli stated "I believe in the phrase 'Carpe Diem.' This is the window of opportunity for hospitalists across the country to claim a vital area of patient care that needs a fresh approach to management."[11] Within the text of this supplement is a clear statement reflecting the failure of anesthesia to fulfill the need for preoperative and postoperative medical management of complex surgical patients, which provides an opportunity for internal medicine–trained surgical hospitalists to fill this void. Whether one disagrees with the premise proposed in this and other publications that internal medicine training provides the best individuals to assume comanagement responsibilities with surgeons and to assume the major role in providing preoperative preparation and postoperative care, it is clearly evident that economic and social considerations have often mitigated against an increased presence of anesthesiologists outside the operative room and out-of-OR anesthetic areas.

Additional training in general internal medicine during anesthesia residency would also strengthen the role of anesthesiologists in preoperative and postoperative assessment and management of patients. It might also help delineate more clearly the distinctions between anesthesiologists and nonphysician anesthesia providers in the OR. With such additional training, the anesthesiologists' role might even evolve further, creating a new subspecialty, the surgical hospitalist. Functioning in this role, the anesthesiologist would allow surgeons to perform surgery without trying to manage patient problems remotely from the OR, facilitate patient care, and ensure that many of the goals and mandates set by the hospital, regulatory agencies and insurers were met. Anesthesiologists with this extended training would be ideally suited for this task because in contrast to most internists, they already understand surgical procedures. Anesthesiologists are also adept at many of the acute issues that are unique to surgical patients, such as fluid, respiratory, and hemodynamic management.

Anesthesiologists assuming a larger role in perioperative medicine and functioning as consultant are not new ideas, although expanding this to that of a surgical hospitalist may be. Numerous articles have been written advocating that anesthesiologists assume a broader role as perioperative physicians, although these articles usually limit the future to preoperative assessment, postoperative care in the postanesthesia care unit and ICU, and acute and chronic pain management.[8] Some of the push in this direction comes from the recognition that as anesthetic drugs, preoperative preparation, and surgical techniques continue to improve, the skills required to anesthetize patients safely in the OR may become more technical than medical.[6] There are exceptions, such as transesophageal echocardiography, which requires both technical skill and understanding of cardiac anatomy, physiology, and pathophysiology, but such examples are the exception rather than the rule. Why then does not the anesthesiologist community embrace a paradigm change to broader participation in the general care of surgical patients? Putatively, this is because of (1) lower reimbursement, (2) limited interest or motivation among anesthesiologists to assume the role of a medical consultant or get involved in the management of surgical patients throughout their hospitalization, and (3) the decreased predictability and greater demand on their time that is required for consultation or direct patient management. There is also a segment of the anesthesiologist community that is confident that the OR will remain the mainstay of practice and that reimbursement will remain relatively stable.[10] There are those who believe, however, that if the profession does not evolve, it cannot survive.[6,12,13] Considering the evolution in the last 40 or so years, the latter possibility seems more likely.

In the past, most surgical patients were admitted to hospitals at least a day before surgery and remained for days following surgery. Anesthesiologists often performed preoperative assessments of the patients whom they themselves would anesthetize the night before surgery, anesthetized them, and sometimes followed them through the recovery room. Those who required intensive care, often for prolonged mechanical ventilation, went to surgical ICUs. These ICUs were often staffed and managed by anesthesiologists, especially in training programs, although the surgeon and surgical residents usually assumed primary responsibility. As outpatient and same-day surgery became more common, it became logistically difficult for an anesthesiologist both to perform the preoperative evaluation and to provide the anesthesia for the same patient. Assessment on the day of surgery led to cancellations and delays to evaluate and resolve medical problems.[14] Several different approaches to solving this problem evolved. Some departments have developed preoperative clinics, staffed and in some cases directed by anesthesia faculty with residents present for education and certified registered nurse anesthetists in various roles including parity with the anesthesiologist. Another tack was for surgeons to refer patients to internists or other consultants for evaluation and to gain "clearance" for surgery with the anesthesiologist seeing the patient on the day of surgery. Although there has been growth in both approaches, it seems that the consultant approach is increasing more rapidly. For example, currently, many of the preoperative guidelines, publications, and textbooks come from internal medicine and its subspecialties with minimal if any involvement from anesthesiologists.[15–18]

With the scourge of poliomyelitis and accompanying respiratory failure in the early 1950s anesthesiologists assumed a major role on providing ventilatory support in specialized units in North America and Europe. This involvement, accompanied by the recognition of the expertise provided through anesthesia training in respiratory physiology and support and led to the beginnings of meaningful contributions by anesthesiologists as ICUs began to appear. One of the first true multidisciplinary ICUs treating a wide variety of critically ill patients was established in Denmark in 1953. Since that time critical care has been a part of many academic anesthesiology programs, but this too is changing. Initially, the role of the anesthesiologist in ICUs was primarily as a consultant in ventilator and hemodynamic management. In some hospitals anesthesiologists also served as the administrative directors of the ICUs, but in general patients were admitted to the surgeon and in large part managed by the surgical residents. Although these functions have not changed in many ICUs, the surgical presence in teaching hospitals has diminished because of the limitations in resident hours, increasing surgical residency caseload requirements, and greater pressure to generate income. Relative to billing for medical management, remuneration for surgical procedures are generally greater, require much less time, and have far less arcane documentation requirements because of global surgical fees. Consequently, surgeons may not take the time to bill for management of their patients' medical conditions that are unrelated to the procedure itself (eg, diabetes, hypertension) because such billing requires detailed notes and learning complex documentation requirements. Instead, they may delegate medical management to consultants who bill for these aspects of care. This may actually be economically more efficient for surgeons if the time gained is used for surgery. This is especially true for ICU care, where the highest level of billing is time-based, requiring a minimum of 30 minutes per patient.

An alternate model is the closed ICU in which patients are admitted to an ICU physician, in some cases an anesthesiologist, who becomes the primary physician while the patient remains in the ICU. Although this model is used in some surgical ICUs, especially those catering to trauma, it is more common for medical patients admitted to medical ICUs and coronary care units, with pulmonologists or cardiologists assuming the role of the primary physician for the patients in the ICU. Rarely, anesthesiologists are the admitting physicians in a closed medical or medical-surgical ICU. These anesthesiologists often have board certification in both internal medicine and anesthesiology.

Regardless of their exact role, many critical care anesthesiologists have evolved beyond the early days of ventilator and hemodynamic management to complete patient care including infection, nutrition, wound management, endocrine issues, and so forth. Providing this level of care often requires a broader knowledge of general medicine than is mandated by current anesthesia residency requirements. Although internists and medicine subspecialists gain exposure to these areas as part of their training, they generally lack experience and in-depth knowledge of many facets relevant to the care of surgical patients (eg, what actually occurs in the OR, anesthetic management, understanding of surgical procedures, pain management, the impact of anesthetics on patients, or even interpreting the anesthetic record). Nonetheless, internists, especially those trained in pulmonary critical care, are playing an increasing role in the ICU management of surgical patients, serving in capacities ranging from routine consultants to assuming primary responsibility for patient care. **Table 1** shows that over the last 7 years whereas the number of anesthesiologists taking critical care fellowships is flat or decreasing, the number of internists has increased by about 40%, and is now 17 times greater than those entering from anesthesiology. The number of surgeons entering critical care fellowships also consistently exceeds anesthesiologists, albeit by a much smaller number. These trends are also reflected in the decrease in the already small and nonincreasing number of programs offering anesthesia critical care fellowships compared with the larger and growing number of programs, especially in medicine but also in surgery.

In contrast to critical care, anesthesiology held a commanding lead in pain medicine, although the numbers did not increase from 2000 to 2004. There were 230 filled positions from 99 programs in 2000 to 2001 when it was the only Accreditation Council for Graduate Medical Education accredited program, whereas in 2004 to 2005 there were 237 filled positions in 97 programs. In contrast, in 2004 to 2005 there were no fellows in the only two pain management programs in neurology, none in the sole program in psychiatry, and 17 fellows in eight programs in physical medicine and rehabilitation. Pain medicine has blossomed since then becoming a multidisciplinary fellowship including anesthesiology, neurology, physical medicine and rehabilitation, and psychiatry with 313 filled positions in 92 programs. Although these data are not broken down by discipline, because specialties other than anesthesiology before the formation of combined programs had very few filled positions, it seems likely that most still come from anesthesiology.

From the data in **Table 1**, it is clear that interest in critical care in anesthesiology is not growing, whereas internal medicine is becoming dominant. Is this important? According to the Report From the Task Force on Future Paradigms of Anesthesia Practice,[3] anesthesiologists must increase their involvement in critical care if their role in perioperative medicine is to grow. Although this is necessary, it is not sufficient. Given the increasing numbers of hospitalists graduating from internal medicine programs and the growing involvement of medicine-trained physicians in preoperative evaluation and critical care, unlike pain medicine where anesthesiologists seem firmly imbedded, to gain a significant role in perioperative care two questions need to be answered: what is the added value of anesthesiologists in perioperative medicine compared with physicians trained in internal medicine and its subspecialties; and does this model

Table 1 Data from Accreditation Council for Graduate Medical Education Web site				
	Anesthesiology	Medicine	Pulmonary Medicine	Surgery
2000–2001				
No. of programs	56	24	116	67
No. of filled positions	111	156	857	110
2004–2005				
No. of programs	49	32	123	85
No. of filled positions	53	154	1098	119
2007–2008				
No. of programs	50	30	130	88
No. of filled positions	82	165	1262	142

extend to the OR (ie, should anesthesiologists be consultants in the OR generally leaving the actual delivery of anesthesia to nonphysician providers)? The answer to the first question is that there is added value in the experience in the management of patients during and at least immediately after surgery. The answer to the second question is that it is consistent for the consultant model to extend to the OR. Rather than trying to make distinctions between physician and nonphysician delivery of anesthesia, the anesthesiologist would become primarily a consultant drawing on the greater exposure in both basic sciences and non–anesthesia-related clinical practice afforded through medical school and resident training. This should not mean that anesthesia residencies need to de-emphasize experience in the actual delivery of anesthesia, because this is vital for consulting with and providing oversight for nonphysician anesthesia providers. It does mean, however, that residencies need to be extended by perhaps a year to provide more knowledge and experience in general patient care. As a concrete example, consider the prospect of deep sedation for colonoscopy of an adult with congenital cardiac lesions. Understanding the anatomy of the lesions and cardiovascular and respiratory physiology, the anesthesiologist should be able to synthesize the potential risks of hemodynamic changes, choose the safest drugs, and anticipate appropriate treatments should adverse events occur. It is unlikely that this could be achieved without the education in hemodynamics and cardiac physiology that is received in medical school and residency. Moreover, the OR experience in interpreting and managing hemodynamics, titrating drugs, and in transesophageal echocardiography is invaluable in managing such a patient and is unlikely to be matched by a nonphysician provider or a physician who has not had training in anesthesiology.

Examples like this showing added value for anesthesiologists compared with internists, medicine subspecialists, and nonphysician anesthesia providers are at the core of the debate on the future of anesthesiologists as perioperative physicians. To continue to develop and expand the perioperative role anesthesiologists must have a knowledge base at least comparable with nonanesthesiologist physicians who are increasingly providing perioperative assessment and management. One clear example of a potentially powerful foray of anesthesiologists into perioperative care is the evaluation and management of cardiac surgical patients. The Departments of Anesthesiology at Stanford University and Anesthesiology Pain and Perioperative Medicine at Brigham and Women's Hospital have developed innovative combined programs in cardiac anesthesiology and critical care. Graduates of these programs are exceptionally well equipped to provide a continuum of care for these patients, including preoperative assessment, OR anesthesia, and ICU management. The in-depth knowledge of pharmacology, anesthesia, cardiac surgical procedures, intraoperative management, transesophageal echocardiography, and the perioperative experience gained in the ICUs and in pain management that is part of the anesthesiologist's training provides a considerable advantage over physicians trained only in medicine and medicine subspecialties in the perioperative assessment and management of such patients.

Recognizing the importance of the expanding role of anesthesiologists in critical care and that anesthesia training should at least ensure that all anesthesiologists have at a minimum some ability to provide care for the critically ill patient beyond the administration of anesthesia, the American Board of Anesthesiologists (ABA) initiated the requirement for 2 months of ICU training in 1983. In 1985, anesthesia gained accreditation status for Critical Care Fellowship Programs and in 1986 offered ABA certification for this subspecialty, the first by the ABA. More recently and now with a 4-year continuum for anesthesia training, time in the ICU has been expanded to 4 months. Some have suggested that anesthesia training be expanded such that all trainees finish with a full year of critical care and be eligible for both critical care medicine and anesthesiology certification, similar to that required by many pulmonary medicine programs.

With respect to preoperative assessment, why should an anesthesiologist request "clearance" for surgery from an internist or medicine specialist? Even more concerning, why should a surgeon make this request when the anesthesiologist should be in a better position to make such assessments because nonanesthesiologist consultants seldom know what actually transpires during anesthesia? Despite the increase in required critical care months in anesthesiology residencies, the depth and breadth of exposure and education in the general medical assessment and management of patients is very limited. Yet, is not the use of consultants for "clearance" an abrogation of the anesthesiologists' responsibilities in patient assessment? Although consultants can be very valuable, should not the request, if needed, be generated by an anesthesiologist accompanied with a specific question for the consultant?

What would be required for anesthesiologists to become dominant in perioperative medicine or to assume a new role as surgical hospitalists? First, it would certainly require additional training in internal medicine. This would likely require another year with a specialized design, reducing the number of ambulatory clinics required in medicine residencies and interspersing the first year of anesthesia residency with the second year of medicine. The ABA had agreed to a combined internal medicine–anesthesiology program conceived at Boston's Brigham and Women's Hospital after which graduates would be board eligible in medicine and anesthesia critical care. Unfortunately, despite support from the Department of Medicine and the ABA, the proposal was rejected by the American Board of Internal Medicine. Perhaps a more realistic approach is to construct a fellowship in perioperative medicine with the possible option to extend it to include a surgical hospitalist fellowship. Alternately, the latter could be a separate fellowship. Both could include critical care and acute pain management. Another, perhaps more productive approach is to follow the lead set by pain management fellowships, creating combined fellowships drawing from anesthesiology, surgery, and medicine. Even if this occurred, however, would residents entering anesthesia programs have any interest in such programs? Judging from the small number entering anesthesiology critical care fellowships, the answer is probably not.

Even without the development of such fellowships, at a minimum more attention could be devoted to the construct of the clinical base year of anesthesia training: the internship. The Resident Review Committee for anesthesia training, the arm of the Accreditation Council for Graduate Medical Education, has proposed that anesthesia programs assume far greater responsibility for the construct of the clinical base year to provide more uniformity and relevance to the nonanesthesia portion of the training. This was done to help ensure that the out-of-OR part of the training is more oriented to the expectations of the anesthesia perioperative physician. These 12 months, if properly supervised, could provide much of the needed experience added to that gained in medical school to prepare the anesthesiologists the means to act as a true colleague and consultant in a comanagement role with the surgeon.

If fellowships or more radical changes in anesthesiology residencies are to be implemented, however, what are the major obstacles to recruiting anesthesiologists into such programs? As noted, such changes in paradigm for anesthesiologists require

1. Cooperation from the American Boards of Internal Medicine, Surgery, and Anesthesiology
2. Major modifications in the anesthesia curriculum if this training were incorporated into anesthesiology residencies

3. Development of a new subspecialty if this were to occur as a fellowship
4. A different mindset among medical students entering anesthesiology residencies
5. Reimbursement and lifestyle comparable with OR-based anesthesiologists

Billing for consulting and hospital care services can use standard inpatient CPT codes as is done in ICUs. Patients could be admitted to an anesthesiologist on a surgical hospitalist service with the surgeon still billing a modified global fee. Different models could be used for different services. Nonetheless, remuneration is unlikely to match that of today's OR-based anesthesia practice. Hospitals might be willing, however, partially to subsidize salaries and overhead as they currently do for some preoperative clinics and hospitalists. The rationale is better and more efficient care. Improvements in metrics that affect hospital reimbursement, such as hospital length of stay, and conditions acquired during hospitalization, such as urinary tract infections, central line bloodstream infections, and skin breakdown, have already impacted on hospital reimbursement and might provide an incentive for hospitals to contribute to such programs.

Whether any or all of this is a pipe dream or actually comes to pass remains to be seen. However, given the improvements in drugs, anesthesia delivery systems, preoperative preparation, and the increasing push towards physician independence of nonphysician anesthesia practitioners to remain a vibrant and viable profession anesthesiologists must not only recapture their traditional perioperative roles but also evolve beyond this into new areas that emphasize value of having physicians trained in OR patient management practicing medicine outside of the traditional OR roles.

Regardless, currently anesthesia critical care training provides experience in the initial assessment of patients, which is invaluable when outpatients are seen for the first time for a procedure outside of the OR. Moreover, It exposes anesthesiologists to the initial assessment and management of conditions that usually have been carefully evaluated and resolved by the time a patient goes to the OR. However, anesthesiology critical care fellowships provide some but not all of this requisite knowledge and experience with gaps that should be closed with additional training in internal medicine. Anesthesiologists with such training should be able to fill a niche in the assessment and management of out-of-OR procedures that are becoming increasingly frequent and cannot be adequately met without training in anesthesiology. Moreover, such individuals should be well suited not just to be perioperative physicians but also to manage surgical patients throughout their hospital stay.

REFERENCES

1. Grant PJ, Wesorick DH. Perioperative medicine for the hospitalized patient. Med Clin North Am 2008;92:325–48.
2. Joshi GP. The anesthesiologist as perioperative physician. Amer Soc Anesth Newsletter 2008;72(4):6–7.
3. Miller RD. Report from the task force on future paradigms of anesthesia practice. Amer Soc Anesth Newsletter 2005:69.
4. Modell JH. Assessing the past and shaping the future of anesthesiology: the 43rd Rovenstine lecture. Anesth 2005;102:1050–7.
5. Johnstone RE. Future of anesthesia practice: views from the conference on practice management. Amer Soc Anesth Newsletter 2005:71.
6. Roy RC, Calicott RW. Anesthesia practice models, perioperative risk and the future of anesthesiology. Amer Soc Anesth Newsletter 2005:71.

7. O'Connor MF, Maccioli GA. The changing face of anesthesiology and perioperative medicine. Amer Soc Anesth Newsletter 2008:72.
8. Adesanya AO, Joshi GP. Hospitalists and anesthesiologists as perioperative physicians: are their roles complementary? Proc (Bayl Univ Med Cent) 2007;20: 140–2.
9. Rock P. The future of anesthesiology is perioperative medicine. Anesthesiol Clin North America 2000;18(3):495–513.
10. Bacon DR, Lema MJ. From the crow's next. Amer Soc Anesth Newsletter 2006; 70(4).
11. Merli G. Perioperative medicine: a fundamental facet of our identity. From perioperative care a special supplement to the official publication of the Society of Hospital Medicine; 2005:4.
12. Miller RD. Sugammadex: an opportunity to change the practice of anesthesiology? Anesth Analg 2007;104(3):477–8.
13. Miller RD. Perspective of a nonintensivist: why critical care medicine is important to the future of our specialty. Amer Soc Anesth Newsletter 2006;70(4).
14. Correll DJ, Bader AM, Hull MW, et al. Value of preoperative clinic visits in identifying issues with potential impact on operating room efficiency. Anesthesiology 2006;105(6):1254–9 [discussion: 6A].
15. Brett AS. Coronary assessment before noncardiac surgery: current strategies are flawed. Circulation 2008;117:3145–51.
16. Fleisher LA, Beckman JA, Brown KA, et al. ACC/AHA 2007 guidelines on perioperative cardiovascular evaluation and care for noncardiac surgery: executive summary: a report of the American College of Cardiology/American Heart Association Task Force on practice guidelines (Writing Committee to Revise the 2002 Guidelines on Perioperative Cardiovascular Evaluation for Noncardiac Surgery): developed in collaboration with the American Society of Echocardiography, American Society of Nuclear Cardiology, Heart Rhythm Society, Society of Cardiovascular Anesthesiologists, Society for Cardiovascular Angiography and interventions, society for vascular medicine and biology, and society for vascular surgery. Circulation 2007;116(17):1971–96.
17. Gregoratos G. Current guideline-based preoperative evaluation provides the best management of patients undergoing noncardiac surgery. Circulation 2008; 117(24):3134–44 [discussion: 3134].
18. Mukherjee D, Eagle KA. Perioperative cardiac assessment for noncardiac surgery: eight steps to the best possible outcome. Circulation 2003;107(22): 2771–4.

Anesthesiology and Competitive Strategy

Wendy L. Gross, MD, MHCM[a],*, Barbara Gold, MD[b]

KEYWORDS

- Competitive strategy • Business model
- Health care economics • Market forces
- Finance • Reimbursement

Whether we like it or not, medicine is big business. The argument is sometimes made that standard management strategies from the business world do not apply to medicine because the economics and practice of medicine are unique—driven by science and rapid rates of change. But an exploding knowledge base, light-speed technological development, and ever-changing reimbursement schemes are not exclusive to medicine and health care. Some fundamental principles of finance, business management, and strategic development have evolved to deal with problems of rapid change. These principles do apply to modern medicine. The business side of anesthesia practice is off-putting to many clinicians. However, knowledge of the market forces at play can help enhance patient care, improve service, expand opportunities, and extend the perimeter of the discipline. The mission and current market position of anesthesiology practice are considered here.

ANESTHESIOLOGY: THEORY OF THE BUSINESS

Successful companies are built upon a "Theory of the Business"[1] based upon market assessment, a mission statement, and commitment to the "core competencies"[1] required for execution of the mission. Any such theory must be dynamic. Constant reassessment of the business environment, the company mission, and its capacity to succeed in that mission is essential to continued success. The economic landscape is littered with businesses unable to adapt to a changing environment. Consider, for example, the unexpected difficulties of GM, AT&T, Sears, IBM, Woolworth, and Lehman Brothers. As that short list implies, not every business succeeds in the effort to

[a] Department of Anesthesia, Perioperative and Pain Medicine, Brigham and Women's Hospital, 75 Francis Street, Boston, MA 02115, USA
[b] Department of Anesthesiology, University of Minnesota Medical Center, Minneapolis, MN, USA
* Corresponding author.
E-mail address: wgross@partners.org (W.L. Gross).

Anesthesiology Clin 27 (2009) 167–174
doi:10.1016/j.anclin.2008.10.013
1932-2275/08/$ – see front matter © 2009 Elsevier Inc. All rights reserved.

adapt to change, but many others have met the challenges, and with appropriate modifications have flourished.

Businesses fail because their activities and decision trees do not reflect market values and behaviors. Their core competencies are either eroded or are no longer appropriate for the needs of current and potential customers, or for a new context or market which is not perceived to be significant.

The core competencies of anesthesiologists include the assessment of medical risks, the development and execution of customized anesthesia plans, and the performance of postoperative care regimens in recovery areas and intensive care units. Providers of anesthesia services in the operating room (OR) are essential for their ability to safely and controllably support the physiologic processes of patients undergoing surgical procedures. Anesthesia care teams are recognized for possessing those competencies and have been highly valued for that reason.

Do our assumptions, current values, and core competencies effectively translate to environments outside the OR, where the procedure, and the degree of physiologic trespass, may be very different, and where the innovative character of the procedure may generate challenges that have not been encountered? Is the value of an anesthesia care team outside of the OR sufficiently high for proceduralists to justify waiting for, or negotiating with, an anesthesia team? Alternatively, given the noninvasive nature of many new procedures, the "disruptive technology"[2] of newer drugs, enhanced monitoring, and drug administration devices, will interventionists forge ahead with anesthesia on their own, preferring to rely on the availability of code teams in the event of an unanticipated problem?

Although noninvasive procedures do not require incisions, they often carry equal or higher risk potentials than similarly focused surgeries. There is insistent demand for rapid turnover and high throughput because investment in new technology is expensive and adequate return on investment requires that interventionalists perform a high volume of procedures. The target patient population is somewhat unpredictable and includes many with significant comorbidities who are deemed too sick for surgery. A significant proportion is not evaluated before the procedure. The variability in patient condition and procedural complexity makes rational and preemptive allocation of anesthesia resources difficult. Anesthesiologists' well-honed risk assessment skills should be applied to the triage of patients undergoing non-OR procedures.

If scheduling was filtered by anesthesiologists, relatively straightforward patients and uncomplicated procedures could probably be delegated safely to skilled sedation nurses operating under an anesthesiologist's supervision. Patients with extensive comorbidities or complex procedures should be consistently assigned to an anesthesia care team. The clinician's level of training should be matched to the difficulty of the medical problem. Highly skilled practitioners should not be forced "down market."

The most favorable condition would be for the highest level of evaluation to be applied to all patients by anesthesiologists who can integrate their special competences in perioperative assessment with a thorough understanding of (1) the procedures being performed and (2) the technologies being applied. This requires that anesthesiologists make an effort to communicate with interventionists, and vice versa, and endeavor to learn the intricacies of new, noninvasive approaches to medical problems.

For patients undergoing multiple procedures during one hospitalization, pre- and postprocedure care recommendations could be formulated by anesthesiologists working as perioperative physicians in a surgical hospitalist role. Adequate preparation for, and timing of, procedures to be performed would minimize length of stay and maximize quality of care. By following the recommendations of anesthesiologists as surgical hospitalists, proceduralists and ancillary personnel would avoid the precipitous situation of caring for patients with multiple unrecognized risk factors, exposing both patients and providers to unnecessary risk. This is just one example of how anesthesiology's, or any other industry's, theory of business needs to be continually re-examined so that it fits the needs of a changing environment.

Market Forces and Analysis

Strategic planning for changing environmental (ie, market) forces is a key element of survival in the business world, and in medicine as well. In his classic analysis, Porter[3,4] identifies five market forces that must be assessed in developing an effective competitive strategy. These are generated by (1) buyers, (2) suppliers (3) barriers to entry, (4) the threat of substitutes, and (5) potential rivalries. Understanding and addressing these forces and their impact upon anesthesia services in the non-OR environment provides a useful framework for further analysis.

Buyers
Who are the buyers of non-OR services and how powerful are they? They are hospitals, practitioners and patients seeking anesthesia services outside of the operating room. A powerful buying group, by definition, is able to demand higher quality or increased quantity of service or product at a lower price. Powerful buying groups are those with a large volume of business and are most successful with products that are easily standardized, enabling the buyer to shop around when the quality of the product is not paramount. Buying groups are most powerful when they can easily "backward integrate" (ie, perform the service themselves, as in nurse-administered sedation). Clearly, with respect to anesthesia services, quality *is* critical and the product is not easily standardized. This is not always understood by proceduralists. The threats of backward integration and of potentially high and increasing volume are readily apparent to the knowledgeable observer.

Suppliers
Suppliers within an industry are persons or organizations providing the resources needed to accomplish the industry's mission. If there are only a few suppliers providing highly specialized resources, and the cost of switching suppliers is considerable, then suppliers occupy a dominant position in the business under consideration. The supply of specialized personnel to match the medical acuteness of the situation is critical in non-OR anesthesia. The suppliers of personnel include anesthesia training programs, anesthesia departments and groups, and hospital nurse or certified registered nurse anesthetist (CRNA) pools. The challenge is to reach agreement about the needs of the patient and to make proceduralists aware of the level of need before disaster threatens. Financial and time constraints are not always absent from such considerations. A shortage of fully qualified anesthesia personnel for staffing non-OR procedures adequately will surely lower the switching costs to nonanesthesia personnel. This is not likely to be in the profession's, or the patient's, best interest.

Quality of service
Quality of service is hard to quantify unless there is a catastrophic outcome. Small problems are rarely documented and the costs are poorly or infrequently tabulated. These problems include longer stays in recovery areas, unanticipated hospital admissions, and nonreimbursement of Centers for Medicare and Medicaid Services (CMS) defined "never-events." Electronic databases and ongoing required quality assessments by third party payers are likely to improve the situation if the necessary information is recorded and available.

Barriers to entry

Barriers to entry within anesthesia practice are considerable but not insurmountable and include the constant push for the use of propofol by individuals not skilled in airway management and the debate over the boundary between deep sedation and general anesthesia. As drugs, monitoring, and skills among providers who are not anesthesiologists improve, the barriers to entry in the non-OR environment will likely decrease, and thereby the opportunity for anesthesia personnel to contribute to the care of these patients must also decrease. This will diminish the value of the anesthesia service within the larger organization. Rather than rely on the protective character of barriers to entry, the challenge is to consider new roles for anesthesiologists and to determine how best to participate in the care of these patients so that all parties are valued. As some barriers are lowered, others arise. New skills will be required as our core competencies are challenged in novel ways. Our roles as integrators of services and supervisors of procedure units may grow, and we will be asked to exploit our medical backgrounds more fully as proceduralists become more and more specialized in the foci of interventions they perform.

Substitution

Another important market force is substitution. In non-OR anesthesia practice, one already existing substitution is the use of a sedation nurse supervised by a proceduralist instead of an anesthesiologist. Although the anesthesia community may bristle at such a prospect, if there is no anesthesia care team available and the procedure, in the eyes of the proceduralist, requires only a little sedation, then why not substitute other willing and available providers for the anesthesiologist? Recent technological innovations purporting to incorporate combination drug administration and monitoring devices could, in principle, replace human providers of sedation or anesthesia altogether. The danger is that perceived substitutes may not be true substitutes. In this context, marketing, effective mutual communication and transfer pricing become important issues.

Rivalry within the industry

The fifth market force that all industries must consider is rivalry within the industry. For example, a hospital may decide to contract with an outside anesthesia provider to meet the needs of non-OR anesthesia, if that seems financially and medically prudent. In some ways, proceduralists themselves are rivals, since they seek to develop pain-free procedures requiring little, if any, intervention by anesthesiologists or ancillary personnel. However, as nontrivial risk will always be present in such procedures, the practice of assuming no need for anesthesia services seems unlikely to be in the best interest of patients. This recognition sets the stage for rivalry and competition among anesthesia groups and interventionalists. Competition can be advantageous to the consumer, in this case the hospital, but it can generate disorganization and inconsistency; which results in potentially poor quality care and lowered reimbursement. The development of an informed competitive strategy will be stimulated by (1) analysis of market forces, (2) consideration of anesthesia's theory of business, and (3) consideration of business theory adaptation.

STRATEGIC PRIORITIES FOR THE FUTURE

The anesthesia community is aware that it faces a compelling need to extend its footprint beyond the limits of the OR. To include procedural areas within the perimeter of our practice we may need to establish a new model of service delivery. Not only are new markets emerging, but the financial rules are changing. We are in danger of allowing our core competencies to fall out of step with current opportunities, and of seeing our theory of the business grow outdated. Disruptive technologies and noninvasive approaches to surgical problems threaten to change the standards for where, and how, surgical and percutaneous interventions are performed.

Anesthesiology revolutionized safety and the scope of practice within the OR, and the potential exists for us to do the same outside the OR. The time-honored role of anesthesiologists in the OR may soon be supplanted, or expanded, by anesthesiologists serving as critical-care providers inside and outside of the intensive care unit (ICU), as sedation supervisors, and as out-of-OR innovators. If we ignore these trends and the emerging market structure, we abdicate our responsibility to patients and to medicine. We need to examine where we stand at this moment and where we want to be with regard to the productivity and the sustainability of anesthesiology as a medical sub-specialty. What are the components of effective strategy?

OPERATIONAL EFFECTIVENESS

Operational effectiveness is one component of competitive strategy and is necessary in order for the provision of anesthesia services to be profitable. Although operational effectiveness embraces all forms of efficiency, it also implies innovativeness and the ability to manage a wider spectrum of activities than the competition. Who or what, then, is "the competition?" For anesthesia services outside of the OR, the competition consists of (1) medical proceduralists who believe they don't need an anesthesiologist, (2) other non anesthesiologists, (3) sedation providers, and (4) companies that design and produce machinery capable of administering drugs and interpreting monitoring apparatuses. "Innovativeness" means providing flexible, adaptive services that can yield recognizably better outcomes. Better outcomes will eventually be more favorably reimbursed.

Better outcomes are defined by quality data and other forms of evidence; therefore, conscientious record keeping and data analysis must become an essential element of operations. Operational effectiveness is achieved by well-planned resource management using adequate management information systems, by the provision of innovative services, and by high-quality database maintenance and analysis. It also requires foresight and close attention to the changing details of the practice on the part of leadership because it serves as an instrument with which to maintain necessary standards and to advance the perimeters of performance. The performance frontier is dependent upon productivity and is constantly shifting as technology develops and new markets emerge. The frontier cannot move if ongoing resource management allows or even encourages operational ineffectiveness.

COSTS, UNIQUENESS, AND VALUE ADDED

Competitive strategy development is about maintaining and delivering a unique or a higher quality of service than the competition. Anesthesiologists clearly have the edge in flexibility, expertise, and medical knowledge for delivery of a superior anesthesia product outside the OR. Strategic edge can be maintained only if services are provided differently, better, and more cost-effective than the existing, or potential, competition can provide them.

Is maintaining the edge possible, given current reimbursement strategies, bundling tactics, and potential CMS reforms? If cost accounting is properly performed (ie, employing variable rather than full-costing techniques) it becomes clear that the cost of patient care involving an efficiently deployed anesthesiologist is less than the cost imposed on the whole system by those inevitable cases which start with nonanesthesia personnel and end with an urgent and unanticipated call for an anesthesiologist. The expense is enormous for (1) delaying a case, (2) stopping a procedure for inadequate sedation, (3) hospitalizing a patient, and (4) redoing the procedure. The cost of pulling an anesthesiologist from another location is high, but the cost of a bad outcome is far higher.

The institution in which anesthesiologists practice, and the medical and surgical departments they serve, benefit from their services. However, reimbursement to anesthesiologists in non-OR arenas is often inadequate because anesthesiologists can only bill for one case at a time, or cannot bill at all because they are supervising multiple cases. There is no reimbursement for supervising cases attended by sedation nurses or for being available. The benefits of improved quality of care accrue to other departments and to the hospital. In this situation, anesthesia services should be billed as overhead in a step-down fashion, and paid for by departments using the service, just as laundry and electricity costs are assigned proportionally as overhead to all departments using these resources.

RECONCILIATION AND STRATEGIC POSITIONING

Strategic positioning should be based on the needs of customers, potential customers, and market shifts. For example, the variety of anesthesia services must be expanded appropriately to include formulation and oversight of plans for anesthesia administration, when necessary, by nonphysician providers. This amounts to reconciling the theory of the business and revision of core competencies with the results of environmental scanning, context analysis, and other standard tools of market assessment. The customers are not just patients; they are also medical proceduralists and third-party payers. When a large, successful industry gets into trouble it is usually because the assumptions underlying the company's behaviors are inconsistent with reality, or because the original collective learning and production skills necessary for a product with a competitive advantage have been lost or have become obsolete.

In response to the emerging new realities and opportunities, anesthesiologists must revise their core competencies to ensure that noncustomers become customers, because it is not in their interests (with regard to finance or standards of medical care) to remain noncustomers. It may be ideologically preferable for medical proceduralists to perform their interventions independently. However, if we can provide a clearly safer, more comfortable, and more time-efficient environment for their practices, and we have the data to prove that we do, then the value of an anesthesiologist in attendance becomes unmistakable. Not only does it become clear to proceduralists and patients, it also becomes clear to insurance companies, regulatory bodies and government agencies.

FINANCIAL SILOS AND TEAMWORK

Proper strategies can be developed only if goals are consistent with market trends, the budget neutrality of CMS, and the absolute certainty of an increasing insistence upon integrated care by third- party payers. Just as anesthesiology developed specialization within the OR, it is likely to continue to do so with venues outside the OR. Not only will this facilitate the development of specialty-driven innovation, it will also improve site-specific quality and encourage the growth of specialty teams. As bundling becomes standard and integration is expected by insurance companies, anesthesiologists will come to rely on the strength of relationships forged between themselves and medical specialists. These relationships will grow and develop only as medical specialists begin to comprehend the value of anesthesiologists in attendance during their cases. Teamwork and integrated service are critical to drive both improved quality of care and financial success.

Just as surgeons eventually realized that they could not perform a surgery effectively while properly administering anesthesia, medical specialists will also come to understand that as procedures and patients become more complicated, they will have to depend on someone else for the performance of anesthesia; whether that is deep sedation monitored or supervised by an anesthesiologist, or general anesthesia (GA) performed exclusively by an anesthesiologist. This will not happen if the appropriate teams and routinely cooperative relationships are not solidly in place.

Team building requires communication and a common language with a common experience and vocabulary; hence the argument for grouping medical specialists with anesthesiologists who specialize in a specific type of surgery. Often medical specialists perform interventions with the same goal as open surgeries, but they do not have the surgical perspective that many anesthesiologists learn in the OR. Integration of medical and surgical perspectives can be, and has been, exploited for innovative solutions to new problems and to avert calamity outside of the OR. The contributions of cardiac anesthesiologists as a result of their intraoperative and three-dimensional transesophageal echocardiography experience to percutaneous device placement and congenital heart disease cases in the catheterization laboratory (Cath Lab) is a case in point. Similar contributions to ultrasound-guided cases in the endoscopy laboratory and to interventional radiology cases are also possible. Teams bridge reimbursement silos. Integration of reimbursement is coming. Why not be ready for it and organize ourselves preemptively?

SUSTAINABLE STRATEGY: KEY ELEMENTS

The goal of any strategy is to maintain a dynamic and profitable market presence consistent with demand and market growth. Anesthesiologists have two parallel sets of priorities: creating and maintaining a stable but flexible customer base, and achieving financial sustainability.

Operational effectiveness will ensure that appropriate resource allocation permits innovation. Enhanced core competencies resulting from expanded medical training and out-of-OR experience will provide a basis for enrichment of services. Team building will ensure that proceduralists understand the rationale for close cooperation and generate a foundation for revenue sharing and overhead payments. Silo-integration will enhance productivity and quality of care across the board. The overall strategy must be to make our specialty indispensable to noncustomers and potential customers, while enhancing the lives of patients by improving outcomes and stimulating progress.

Our expertise will justify reliable and sustained reimbursement if we have the data to demonstrate the benefit of that presence. Our participation in interventional procedures can stimulate and advance medicine just as our development of the OR environment advanced the practice of surgery. As technology continues to proliferate and diversify, medical specialists will perform many of what are now surgical procedures in noninvasive ways and surgeons will progress to other methods of performing their procedures. Only by pursuing innovation and the building of integrative bridges can anesthesiology hope to survive as a specialty.

Anesthesiology, like other specialties, is at risk. New markets have emerged from advances in basic medical science and the explosion of new technologies. Former noncustomers have become customers. New competition from formerly peripheral personnel and technology is evident, but at the same time, financial disincentives to development are widespread. There is an urgent need for us to engage a broader business-like perspective to reassess our assumptions about the environment, the mission, and the core competencies of our discipline. If we ignore this responsibility, our very status as a medical subspecialty may be threatened. If we accept it, we will be on the front lines as the frontiers of medicine advance.

REFERENCES

1. Drucker Peter. Theory of the business. Harvard Business Review, Sept–Oct 1994.
2. Clayton Christenson. The innovator's dilemma. Harvard Business Review, Sept–Oct 2.
3. Porter M. What is strategy? Harvard Business Review, Nov–Dec 1996.
4. Porter M. How competitive forces shape strategy Harvard Business Review, March/April 1979.

Index

Note: Page numbers of article titles are in **boldface** type.

A

Ablation, catheter, role of out-of-operating room anesthesiologist in, 38
    anesthesia for, 53–54
Accountable care organizations, and improving integration of care in Medicare, 13
Anesthesia, out of operating room, 1–174
    competitive strategy and, **167–174**
        costs, uniqueness, and value added, 171–172
        financial silos and teamwork, 172–173
        operational effectiveness, 171
        reconciliation and strategic positioning, 172
        strategic priorities for the future, 170–171
        sustainable strategy, key points of, 173–174
        theory of business, 167–170
    consultation, communication, and conflict management in, **111–120**
        conflicts in the medical setting, 116–119
        effective consultant, 112–116
    financial and operational analysis of, **17–23**
        differential costing, 18–19
        full costing, 17–18
        management control implications, 20
        more efficient use of resources through operations management, 20–22
        potential consequences of incorrect decisions, 19–20
    for cardiac patients, **29–46**
        electrophysiology interventions, 37–40, **47–56**
        in the cardiac catheterization and electrophysiology laboratories, 30–37, **47–56**
        transesophageal echocardiography, 40–41
    in gastroenterology endoscopy practice, **57–70, 71–85**
        BARRX Medical Halo System, 64
        deep-balloon enteroscopy, 67
        endoscopic mucosal resection/endoscopic submucosal dissection, 64–66
        future directions in endoscopic sedation, 60–61
        gastroenterologist-directed propofol sedation, 59
        high-resolution and magnification endoscopy and chromoendoscopy, 66–67
        managing complications, 81
        medical and legal implications of propofol, 59–60
        medications for, 74–77
        natural orifice translumenal endoscopic surgery, 62–63
        other practical issues, 73–74
        postanesthesia recovery, 81–82
        propofol use in GI endoscopy, 58–59
        role of anesthesiology in, 61–62
        sedation *vs.* anesthesia, 72–73
        sedation/anesthesia for specific procedures, 77–81

Anesthesiology Clin 27 (2009) 175–183
doi:10.1016/S1932-2275(09)00014-7
1932-2275/08/$ – see front matter © 2009 Elsevier Inc. All rights reserved.

Moving?

Make sure your subscription moves with you!

To notify us of your new address, find your **Clinics Account Number** (located on your mailing label above your name), and contact customer service at:

E-mail: elspcs@elsevier.com

800-654-2452 (subscribers in the U.S. & Canada)
314-453-7041 (subscribers outside of the U.S. & Canada)

Fax number: 314-523-5170

Elsevier Periodicals Customer Service
11830 Westline Industrial Drive
St. Louis, MO 63146

*To ensure uninterrupted delivery of your subscription, please notify us at least 4 weeks in advance of move.

Printed and bound by CPI Group (UK) Ltd, Croydon, CR0 4YY

03/10/2024

01040462-0017